Cannabis in Medical Practice

A primer on the endocannabinoid system and herbal therapy for patients and their healthcare professionals

David Bearman, MD, Carolina Nocetti, MD,

Maria Pettinato, RN, PhD, and Angela Bacca

Foreword by Raphael Mechoulam, PhD

All rights reserved. No part of this book may be reproduced or used in any manner without the prior written permission of the copyright owner, except for the use of brief quotations in a book review. To request permissions, contact the publisher at
angela@flowervalley.press

© 2024 David Bearman, MD, Carolina Nocetti, MD, Maria Pettinato, RN, PhD, and Angela Bacca

Edited by Angela Bacca and Amber Finnegan
Cover Design by Jose Luis Cordovez

First paperback edition 2024
ISBN: 979-8-9890163-4-1

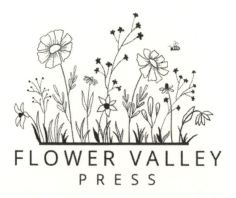

Lompoc, California, United States of America
FlowerValley.Press

This book is dedicated to Dr. Raphael Mechoulam (1930–2023), the researcher who discovered the endocannabinoid system and paved the way for the incorporation of cannabis into clinical practice. It is our hope, as was his, that clinical research continues in earnest and that education about the endocannabinoid system is incorporated into medical school curricula and training for healthcare professionals.

Table of Contents

Foreword	7
Introduction	9
PART I: Cannabis & the Endocannabinoid System	12
History	13
The Human-Cannabis Interaction	19
Constituents & Chemical Characteristics of Cannabis	34
Part II: Cannabis Use & Side Effects	51
Dosing	52
Routes of Administration	61
Metabolism	67
Side Effects of Cannabis	73
Pregnancy	83
Dependence	88
Toxicology	93
Cannabis Use and Driving	94
Part III: Cannabis for Clinicians	97
Introduction to the Medical Use of Cannabis	98
Therapeutic Applications of Cannabis	100
Integrative Medicine	106
Analgesia	110
Autoimmune Diseases	116
Cancer & Symptoms Arising from its Treatment	128
Neurodegenerative & Neurodevelopment-Related Diseases	131
Dr. Bearman's Clinical Standards	146
Part IV: The Future	150
The Future of Cannabis Medicine	151
Glossary	158
Index	166

Foreword

By Raphael Mechoulam, PhD, 1930–2023

Dr. David Bearman is a clinician who became interested in cannabis-based medicine over three decades ago. Very few clinicians at that time knew much about cannabis or were interested in its medical use. For most of them, it was only part of the "horrible" heroin-cocaine-cannabis chemical world, from which physicians had to stay as far away as possible. Dr. Bearman realized that if we knew more about cannabis and its constituents, we could have a new group of valuable drugs. He went to international meetings and was personally associated with researchers. He became one of the first clinicians to use medical cannabis in his practice.

The medical cannabis world has changed immensely since that time. In Israel, about 60,000 Ministry of Health-approved patients are being treated with various medical cannabis drugs. In the United States, cannabidiol (CBD) has been approved as an anti-epileptic drug in certain disease states, while THC is an approved drug for some of the side effects of cancer therapy. In view of the research published on the chemistry, pharmacology, and clinical effects of cannabinoids, it is possible that cannabinoids, in pure form or as well-defined mixtures, will be approved for numerous additional medical conditions. Dr. Bearman realized this therapeutic spring many years ago and has researched, written books, and given talks on the subject.

This book presents the medical cannabinoid field specifically to healthcare professionals and discerning patients. It starts with a fascinating look at history, from its use in China 4,000 years ago through India and the ancient world in the Middle East, the criminalization by a Pope in the fifteenth century, its use by Queen Victoria, and its current use and legal status.

The physiological roles of the endocannabinoid system and the endocannabinoids, as well as the pharmacological effects, are thoroughly described in a style that does not require the use of a medical dictionary. The emphasis of the book is on the medicinal uses of cannabis, the side effects, dependence, and toxicology, as expected from a book for healthcare professionals.

I was particularly impressed by the chapter entitled "Dr. Bearman's Clinical Standards." Based on his medical practice, Dr. Bearman has realized that as medicinal cannabis is not a standard drug, many physicians should take a different approach from those used for other drugs. Dr. Bearman provides a step-by-step in this unusual area of medical practice. I hope and expect that this book will reach a wide audience of medical professionals.

Dr. Mechoulam passed away at the age of 92 in March 2023 before this edition was published. He was the President of the Multidisciplinary Center for Cannabinoid Research at Hebrew University in Jerusalem and is remembered as the "godfather" of modern cannabis science.

Introduction

The campaigns to re-legalize the medicinal use of cannabis in the 1990s were a direct result of the HIV/AIDS epidemic of the 1980s. People were dying, and the medical community had little offer to patients, even to treat the symptoms. Many patients found that cannabis alleviated much of their suffering, although it wasn't curative. The concept of medical use spread beyond HIV/AIDS patients to patients with cancer and other chronic and difficult-to-treat illnesses.

Dennis Peron, the leader of the movement to pass California's groundbreaking Proposition 215, the first state-level law to relegalize cannabis since Prohibition began, famously decried that "all use [of cannabis] is medical" amid criticisms from conservatives and the medical community that these laws were just cover for people who "just wanted to get high."

To medical professionals, the concept that "all use is medical" sounds rather absurd. Medical substances are approved by governments, they are tested in clinical trials, and they come with reliable data about effects, side effects, contraindications, and efficacy. These data points are hard to nail down with cannabis, a botanical substance that, by nature, is not standardized, just like the humans that consume it. The idea that cannabis cannot be medicinal because it is not government-approved exposes a major flaw in our drug approval system. Nature is not standard and no herbal substance in its natural form can meet these requirements.

However, the research done to understand cannabis and how it interacts with the human body led to the identification of an entire physiological system that is critical to human health—the endocannabinoid system. We now understand that cannabis is not the only plant that produces cannabinoids, and cannabinoids are not the only plant compounds that interact with the endocannabinoid system.

Studies on the endocannabinoid system have highlighted the need for allopaths to take a more integrative approach to cannabis and everything else that affects the endocannabinoid system, such as diet, lifestyle, and "alternative" approaches like acupuncture, all of which have been shown to interact with this critical system. More importantly, the reality is that patients are utilizing cannabis and other herbs with or without the help of medical professionals. It is time for doctors, nurses, researchers, and other healthcare professionals to meet the moment.

Using cannabis in clinical care is not an either-or or better-than option; it is a tool that can lead to the discontinuation of treatments with a greater potential to do harm and can empower patients to take control of their own health by providing them with the knowledge they need to utilize it safely.

In this book, we aim to provide doctors, researchers, healthcare professionals, patients, and their caregivers with critical information about cannabis, the endocannabinoid system, and how to consider the addition of herbalism in medical care. Additionally, we aim to demystify cannabis treatment as a panacea and base the conversation about cannabinoid treatment in reality by examining it seriously but not overselling its benefits or efficacy. At the same time, we encourage more honest research about contraindications, side effects, and downsides, as this research, too, has been politicized by Prohibition policies rather than science.

In the context of wellness—of potentially preventing the development of a serious illness, or even simply supplanting the use of alcohol or illicit drugs—is not all use of cannabis then potentially medical? The authors of this book have laid out the body of information so that readers can answer this question for themselves.

This book is meant to be both an easy start guide for patients and their caregivers and an appropriately cited introduction to the therapeutic use of cannabinoids for their doctors. The first part of this book provides the necessary context for current policy through a historical look at the social and political demonization of the cannabis plant that led to its prohibition and continues to stigmatize meaningful research. It introduces the endocannabinoid system, the constituents in cannabis (and many other plants) that interact with it, and the mechanisms of action that cause its effects. The second part of this book provides the necessary information about side effects, potential contraindications, drug interactions, dependence, and toxicology clinicians and patients need to understand to utilize cannabis safely. The third and final part of this book takes a deeper and more scientific approach to examining specific disease states and their interaction with cannabis and the endocannabinoid system. It concludes with standards for clinical incorporation designed by Dr. David Bearman.

Dr. David Bearman, a pioneering California doctor with a rich legacy as a clinician and consultant to state and county governments about substance abuse, wrote the first edition of this book. Subsequent editions were expanded by Angela Bacca, a professional editor and writer specializing in cannabis, herbalism, and alternative healthcare topics and who has used cannabis to treat symptoms of Crohn's Disease for over 20 years. Dr. Maria Pettinato edited and adapted this content to be used as a textbook for a groundbreaking endocannabinoidology class she teaches at the College of Nursing at Seattle University. Dr. Carolina Nocetti, who has led the movement to incorporate cannabis and cannabinoid medicines into clinical practice in Brazil, edited this text and provided new content about treating specific disease states. Each of our unique perspectives was infused into this text to make it useful for medical professionals, students, patients, and their caregivers.

Our goal is to destigmatize cannabis and herbalism in medical care, encourage more medical schools and healthcare training programs to teach about the endocannabinoid system, and empower patients.

We dedicate this book to the "godfather" of endocannabinoid research, Dr. Raphael Mechoulam, whose work has led us all to this place.

Supplemental educational materials are available at www.CannabisInClinicalPractice.com

PART I: Cannabis & the Endocannabinoid System

This section of the book provides background on current cannabis policy through a brief global history of the medicinal use of cannabis. It builds a foundation for clinical incorporation through an overview of the endocannabinoid system, cannabinoids, and other medicinal constituents of cannabis.

History

The cannabis plant originated on the Tibetan plateau in modern-day China approximately thirty-five million years ago.[1] It has been cultivated for at least ten thousand years and is among the oldest cultivated crops in the world. It has been used as a food, **nutraceutical, entheogen, herbal medicine**, and social lubricant for all recorded human history. It evolved and survived by creating cannabinoids and terpenes as a method of self-defense against predators, and today, both have been shown to be essential to its medicinal effects in humans.

Humans have cultivated cannabis for a variety of purposes. **Hemp** varieties were grown for their fibers and seeds to produce paper, fabrics, oils, and food. According to Dr. Richard E. Shultes (1915–2001), from Harvard University, the use of fibers dates back eight thousand years.[2] Varieties typically referred to as marijuana were bred for the sticky cannabinoid and terpene-rich resin produced by their flowers. Cultivated varieties of cannabis, or **"cultivars,"** are distinguished by the unique blends and concentrations of **cannabinoids** and **terpenes** present. International governments have established a threshold of 0.3% of Δ^9-tetrahydrocannabinol (THC) in this plant's composition to distinguish hemp plants from marijuana. This distinction is an arbitrary bureaucratic decision with no basis in current botanical science.[3]

Cannabis has long been used as an analgesic or painkiller. Pain is the most common symptom that drives patients to see a physician. The analgesic properties of cannabis are noted in most, if not all, materia medica ever written. Shen Nung's *Pen Ts'ao Ching* was the earliest known pharmacopeia. It contains ma, cannabis. Shen Nung is considered the Chinese God of Agriculture and possibly the real or mythical Second Emperor of China. The *Pen Ts'ao Ching* was passed on by oral tradition, and it is estimated it originated sometime between 2637 and 2737 BCE.[4]

---

[1] McPartland, J.M., Hegman, W. & Long, T. *Cannabis* in Asia: its center of origin and early cultivation, based on a synthesis of subfossil pollen and archaeobotanical studies. *Veget Hist Archaeobot* 28, 691–702 (2019). https://doi.org/10.1007/s00334-019-00731-8

[2] Schultes, Richard Evans, C. R. B. Joyce and S. H. Curry. "Random thoughts and queries on the botany of cannabis." (1970).

[3] Richard E Schultes. *Random thoughts and queries on the botany of cannabis.* J. & A.1 painkiller. Its analgesic properties are noted in most, if not all, Churchill., 1970. p. 23, 27.

[4] "Medical Cannabis: A Short Graphical History in China." Antique Cannabis Book. Accessed February 1, 2018. http://antiquecannabisbook.com/chap2B/China/China.htm/.

Below is a truncated timeline of the nearly five thousand-year recorded history of the medicinal use of cannabis worldwide:

- **2373 BCE, China**: Listed in the *Pen Ts'ao Ching*, the earliest Chinese materia medica
- **2000 BCE, Egypt**: Prepared as a drink in ancient Thebes
- **500 BCE, Persia**: Used as a sacrament in the practice of Zoroastrianism
- **450 BCE, Scythia**: Inhaled as an intoxicating incense
- **200 BCE, Israel**: Used as a medicine by the Essenes
- **700 CE, Middle East**: Used for divine revelation by Sufi priests
- **1200, Europe**: Banned as a medicine during the Spanish Inquisition
- **1480, Italy**: Criminalized by Pope Innocent VIII
- **1802, France**: Napoleon's soldiers return from Egypt with cannabis samples
- **1835, France**: Club des Haschins established to eat cannabis-infused foods
- **1839, India**: Dr. William O'Shaughnessy researches cannabis in India and reintroduces it to England
- **1850, USA:** Cannabis first listed as a medicine in the United States Pharmacopoeia
- **1892, Great Britain**: Sir William Osler recommends cannabis to treat migraine in medical textbook
- **1895, Great Britain**: Indian Commission for Hemp Drugs: Report details medical uses
- **1914, USA**: Cannabis successfully excluded from the Harrison Narcotics Taxation Act
- **1931, Panama**: Canal Zone Siler report finds cannabis is not habit-forming like opiates and cocaine
- **1937, USA**: The American Medical Association (AMA) testifies against Prohibition in hearings ahead of the passage of the Marihuana Tax Act
- **1942, USA**: Dr. Morris Fishbein, editor of the *Journal of American Medicine*, states cannabis is the best treatment for migraines
- **1961, United Nations**: 186 countries ratify the UN Single Convention on Narcotic Drugs, an international treaty banning coca, opium poppies, and cannabis, and tasks each nation with establishing controlled substance schedules within ten years
- **1969, USA**: The US Supreme Court determines the Marihuana Tax Act is unconstitutional
- **1970, USA**: The Controlled Substances Act passes in accordance with the UN Single Convention on Narcotic Drugs, and marijuana is listed as Schedule I, meaning it has no accepted medical use and a high potential for abuse

- **1978–1991, USA**: The Investigational New Drug program is established to provide a small group of patients with cannabis for therapeutic use
- **1996, USA**: California legalizes medical cannabis
- **1999, Great Britain**: GW Pharmaceuticals starts researching cannabis tincture to create standardized pharmaceutical products
- **1999, USA**: The California State Legislature allocates $9 million for research into the medical uses of cannabis, resulting in the establishment of the Marijuana Research Center at the University of California at San Diego
- **2001, Canada**: Canada becomes the first nation to legalize the medical use of cannabis
- **2005, Canada**: GW Pharmaceuticals' Sativex® is approved for prescription sale by Health Canada
- **2009, USA**: Barack Obama becomes president and appoints Eric Holder as Attorney General. Holder's Department of Justice issues the "Ogden Memo," signaling the administration would not target medical cannabis businesses that comply with state and local laws
- **2010, Great Britain**: GW Pharmaceuticals' Sativex® is approved for prescription sale in the United Kingdom
- **2012, USA**: The non-medical use of cannabis is approved by voter initiative in the states of Washington and Colorado
- **2013, USA**: The Department of Justice issues the "Cole Memo," signaling that the administration would not target adult-use cannabis businesses that comply with state and local laws and put systems in place to ensure products are not accessible to minors and do not cross state lines, among other guidelines
- **2013, Uruguay**: Referencing non-medical legalization in the US as the impetus for breaking the UN Single Convention on Narcotic Drugs, Uruguay becomes the first country to legalize cannabis for non-medical use
- **2017, Canada**: Canada legalizes non-medical use of cannabis
- **2022, USA**: President Joe Biden and Attorney General Merrick Garland announce a review of the scheduling status of cannabis and the release of federal prisoners serving sentences for nonviolent cannabis crimes

At the time of publication, all but three US states have established some form of medical or non-medical commercial cannabis system. Countries throughout Europe and South America have established medical cannabis laws, and countries in North and South America, Europe, Africa, and Asia have legalized non-medical use of cannabis. Modern research is being conducted on the therapeutic properties of cannabis.

A Brief History

Cannabis has a long record of use as a pain reliever.[5] Historically, the analgesic properties of cannabis were recorded in most *materia medica*.[6] The *Pen Ts'ao Ching*, written by Shen Nung—considered the Chinese God of Agriculture and possibly the real or mythical Second Emperor of China—is the oldest known pharmacopeia. Among other herbal medicines, cannabis is cited in this classic work. It is estimated that the *Pen Ts'ao Ching* originated between 2637 and 2737 BCE and was transmitted orally until it was first written down sometime between 300 BCE and 200 BCE.[7] The original text no longer exists, but it is believed to have consisted of three volumes containing 365 entries describing hundreds of medicines, including cannabis.[8]

Over time, the medicinal use of cannabis spread from China, India, and the Middle East to Europe. Hemp was well-known in Europe in the Middle Ages and was used to make beer and as an ingredient in gruel—a common grain breakfast cereal of the time. Nurses and midwives were vilified as witches because they used cannabis to ease the pain of childbirth. In the fifteenth century, Pope Innocent VIII labeled cannabis as an instrument of the devil because of its healing capabilities, eliminating the medical use of cannabis by mainstream physicians in Europe. It may have been as late as the early nineteenth century that the medicinal use of cannabis was reintroduced into Europe by British physician Dr. W.B. O'Shaughnessy.[9]

In the late 1830s, after spending time in India, O'Shaughnessy returned to England, where he worked to establish the telegraph across the country. Upon his return, he reintroduced cannabis to Western medicine. One of the therapeutic attributes he discussed was cannabis's analgesic properties. By the middle of the nineteenth century, cannabis became an important medicine in America. Cannabis medicine caught on quickly and was widely used in many nineteenth-century pain relief preparations. Cannabis was

---

[5] For a more extensive discussion of cannabis for pain see *"The Sacred Plant Plain Book"* which Dr. Bearman was the main medical contributor.

[6] Zuardi AW. *History of cannabis as a medicine: a review.* Braz J Psychiatry. 2006 Jun;28(2):153-7. doi: 10.1590/s1516-44462006000200015. Epub 2006 Jun 26. PMID: 16810401.

[7] *History of Cannabis: Chinese Medicine.* Medical Cannabis - A Short Graphical History. (n.d.). http://antiquecannabisbook.com/chap2B/China/China.htm

[8] França, Inácia & Souza, Jeová & Baptista, Rosilene & Britto, Virgínia. (2008). [Popular medicine: benefits and drawbacks of medicinal plants]. Revista brasileira de enfermagem. 61. 201-8. 10.1590/S0034-71672008000200009.

[9] O'Shaughnessy, William Brooke. "On the preparations of the Indian Hemp, or Gunjah: Cannabis indica their effects on the animal system in health, and their utility in the treatment of tetanus and other convulsive diseases." Provincial Medical Journal and Retrospect of the Medical Sciences 5, no. 123 (1843): 363

prescribed in the 1890s to Queen Victoria of England by her royal physician, Sir J. Russell Reynolds, to relieve pain from menstrual cramps.[10]

Cannabis has been known for centuries as one of the best treatments for the relief of migraine headache symptoms, particularly for relief from accompanying pain and nausea. Sir William Osler, often acknowledged as the founder of modern medicine and one of the four founders of the Johns Hopkins School of Medicine, dubbed cannabis the best migraine treatment in *The Principles and Practice of Medicine* (1892), often considered the first textbook of internal medicine.[11]

From the 1850s to the early 1940s, cannabis was a popular ingredient in both patent and prescription medications. Medicinal cannabis products were manufactured by such well-known pharmaceutical firms as Eli Lilly, Squibb, Merck, Parke-Davis, Sharp and Dohme, and the Smith Brothers. In the 1920s, American physicians wrote three million cannabis-containing prescriptions per year. According to the AMA, use in the late 1930s had decreased because the product was hard to standardize and had a relatively short shelf life.[12] It remained in the United States Pharmacopoeia (USP) until 1942.[13]

However, in 1937, there was yet another attack on cannabis, this time in the form of the Marihuana Tax Act—endorsed by Harry Anslinger, the first head of the Bureau of Narcotics and Dangerous Drugs (BNDD). Over time, the BNDD evolved into what is currently known as the Drug Enforcement Administration (DEA). In that same year, Dr. William C. Woodward, a physician, attorney, chief legal counsel for the American Medical Association, and former president of the American Public Health Association (1914), testified before the House Ways and Means Committee against the Marihuana Tax Act. Dr. Woodward testified that the AMA was aware of the "non-dangerous medical use of cannabis."[14]

---

[10] "History of Marijuana as Medicine - 2900 BC To Present," ProCon. Accessed February 1, 2018. https://medicalmarijuana.procon.org/view.timeline.php?timelineID=000026/.

[11] Osler W, McCrae T. *The Principles and Practice of Medicine*. Appleton: New York, 1915.

[12] Herer, Jack, Jeff Meyers, and Leslie Cabarga. "Cannabis Drug Use in 19th Century America," in the emperor wears no clothes. Ah Ha Pub., 1998. Last modified: February 1, 2018. http://jackherer.com/emperor-3/

[13] Pharmacopeia, United States. "12th rev." Accessed February 1, 2018. http://antiquecannabisbook.com/Appendix/USP1942.htm/

[14] Woodward William C interviewed by The House of Representatives Committee on Ways and Means. Taxation of Marihuana. 1937. http://www.druglibrary.org/Schaffer/hemp/taxact/woodward.htm/.

Dr. Woodward also testified that he had contacted several US government agencies, including the US Public Health Service, the Federal Bureau of Prisons, and the Children's Bureau, and discovered no evidence supporting Harry Anslinger's claims. Woodward claimed Anslinger had no evidence-based facts, all he had were a handful of newspaper clippings. Ignoring Woodward's testimony, Congress approved the Marihuana Tax Act.

Many others have followed Dr. Woodward's lead in pointing out cannabis's incredibly low side effect profile. In 1988, after a two-year rescheduling hearing, the DEA Chief Administrative Law Judge, Francis Young, recommended rescheduling cannabis to Schedule II. Judge Young's finding of fact stated that cannabis, or marijuana as he referred to it, was "one of the safest therapeutic agents known to mankind" and that it was "safer than eating ten potatoes."[15] This recommendation by Judge Young was rejected by George H.W. Bush's DEA Director, John Lawn.

Physicians feel more comfortable recommending or prescribing medication when they understand its mechanisms of action. However, their lack of understanding has not prevented physicians from prescribing many other drugs on the market. The stigma attached to cannabis has created barriers to researching and teaching about the endocannabinoid system and has made it impossible to include cannabis and the endocannabinoid system in the curriculum of medical schools and government-funded clinical research. With the gradual decrease in this stigma and the increase in patient requests, more medical schools are incorporating these subjects into their curriculum and conducting their own research on the medical use of cannabis. The large amount of research published to date provides a scientific basis for teaching, with more than 25,000 articles in peer-reviewed medical journals. The gradual inclusion of these disciplines in medical school curricula is, in turn, increasing the willingness of physicians to take a closer look at this medicine's 4,000-year-old history of use.

---

[15] Drug Enforcement Administration. Young, Francis L. "In the Matter of Marijuana Rescheduling Petition - Opinion and Recommended Ruling, Findings of Fact, Conclusions of Law and Decision of Administrative Law Judge "September 6, 1988.

The Human-Cannabis Interaction

The effects associated with cannabis use depend on the act of its active principles on specific receptors, thus modulating various physiological functions. These receptors are part of a system called the **endocannabinoid system**.

Endocannabinoid System (ECS)

The ECS consists of **endogenous cannabinoids, or endocannabinoids**, compounds made within the human body, and **cannabinoid receptors** found on cells throughout the body that bind with them and cause a wide variety of physiological effects. The ECS acts as a central system for regulating emotional and behavioral responses, as well as social interactions.[16]

The best-known ECS receptors are the cannabinoid receptor type 1 (CB1)[17] and type 2 (CB2)[18], but there are at least four or five other receptors that are currently being studied. Among them are GPR55 and GPR119, PPAR receptors, and some vanilloid receptors.[19,20] The two best-known endocannabinoids are N-arachidonoyl ethanolamide (AEA), more commonly known as **anandamide**, and 2-arachidonoylglycerol (2-AG), which act as endogenous agonists of CB1 and CB2 receptors.[21,22] These ligands are metabolized by their

---

[16] Katona, I., & Freund, T. F. (2012). "Multiple functions of endocannabinoid signaling in the brain." *Annual Review of Neuroscience, 35*(1), 529–558. https://doi.org/10.1146/annurev-neuro-062111-150420

[17] Matsuda, L. A., Lolait, S. J., Brownstein, M. J., Young, A., & Bonner, T. I. (1990). "Structure of a cannabinoid receptor and functional expression of the cloned cDNA." *Nature, 346*(6284), 561–564. https://doi.org/10.1038/346561a0

[18] Munro, S., Thomas, K. L., & Abu-Shaar, M. (1993). "Molecular characterization of a peripheral receptor for cannabinoids." *Nature, 365*(6441), 61–65. https://doi.org/10.1038/365061a0

[19] Di Marzo, V., & Piscitelli, F. (2015). "The Endocannabinoid System and its Modulation by Phytocannabinoids." *Neurotherapeutics, 12*(4), 692–698. https://doi.org/10.1007/s13311-015-0374-6

[20] Cristino, L., Bisogno, T., & Di Marzo, V. (2019). "Cannabinoids and the expanded endocannabinoid system in neurological disorders." *Nature Reviews Neurology*, 16(1), 9–29. https://doi.org/10.1038/s41582-019-0284-z

[21] Devane, W. A., Hanuš, L., Breuer, A., Pertwee, R. G., Stevenson, L., Griffin, G., Gibson, D., Mandelbaum, A., Etinger, A., & Mechoulam, R. (1992). "Isolation and structure of a brain constituent that binds to the cannabinoid receptor." *Science, 258*(5090), 1946–1949. https://doi.org/10.1126/science.1470919

[22] Sugiura, T., Kondo, S., Sukagawa, A., Nakane, S., Shinoda, S., Itoh, K., Yamashita, A., & Waku, K. (1995). "2-Arachidonoylglycerol: a possible endogenous cannabinoid receptor ligand in brain." *Biochemical and Biophysical Research Communications, 215*(1), 89–97. https://doi.org/10.1006/bbrc.1995.2437

degrading enzymes, fatty acid amide hydrolase (FAAH) and monoacylglycerol lipase (MAGL).[23,24,25]

ANANDAMIDE

2-ARACHIDONOYLGLYCEROL (2-AG)

Endocannabinoids anandamide (AEA) and 2-arachidonoylglycerol (2-AG) chemical structures. SOURCE: Dinu, Robert & Popa, Simona & Mota, Maria. (2011). The Role of the Endocannabinoid System in the Pathogeny of Type 2 Diabetes. 10.5772/21304.

Primary Components of the ECS

Main receptors	CB1 and CB2
Other receptors	TRPR1, GPR-18, -55, -119 and PPARS
Endocannabinoid synthesis' enzymes	NAPE-PLD and sn-1 / DAGLs and β
Endocannabinoid degradation enzymes	FAAH and MAGL
ECS receptors' endogenous ligands	AEA and 2-AG

---

[23] Cravatt, B. F., Giang, D. K., Mayfield, S. P., Boger, D. L., Lerner, R. A., & Gilula, N. B. (1996). "Molecular characterization of an enzyme that degrades neuromodulatory fatty-acid amides." *Nature*, 384(6604), 83–87. https://doi.org/10.1038/384083a0

[24] Dinh, T. P., Freund, T. F., & Piomelli, D. (2002). "A role for monoglyceride lipase in 2-arachidonoylglycerol inactivation." *Chemistry and Physics of Lipids*, 121(1–2), 149–158. https://doi.org/10.1016/s0009-3084(02)00150-0

[25] Ligresti, A., De Petrocellis, L., & Di Marzo, V. (2016). "From phytocannabinoids to cannabinoid receptors and endocannabinoids: pleiotropic physiological and pathological roles through complex pharmacology." *Physiological Reviews*, 96(4), 1593–1659. https://doi.org/10.1152/physrev.00002.2016

The elements that integrate the ECS are expressed in different tissues and systems of the human body.[26] CB1 receptors are located, for example, in nervous, hepatic, adipose, vascular, cardiac, reproductive, and bone tissues, with the greatest density being observed in the brain.[27] CB2 receptors are widely expressed in immune system cells but can also be found in other tissues such as nervous tissue or the gastrointestinal tract.[28,29] In general, the stimulation of CB1 receptors is responsible for the **psychotropic** (inebriating) effect of cannabis, while the stimulation of CB2 receptors promotes the reduction of inflammation, decreases tissue damage, and accelerates the regeneration process in several pathological states.[30]

The ECS's broad expression in the human body and its involvement in the modulation of diverse biological functions make it "perhaps the most important physiological system involved in the establishment and maintenance of human health."[31] The ECS is essential for the maintenance of **homeostasis**[32] and is involved in a wide variety of physiological processes, including appetite, analgesia, mood, and memory.[33] In simple terms, the human organism is extremely "friendly" to cannabinoids, both those it produces internally and those that are sourced from plants, primarily cannabis.

---

[26] Mackie, K. (2008). "Cannabinoid Receptors: Where They are and What They do." *Journal of Neuroendocrinology, 20*(s1), 10–14. https://doi.org/10.1111/j.1365-2826.2008.01671.x

[27] Mechoulam, R., & Parker, L. A. (2013). "The endocannabinoid system and the brain." *Annual Review of Psychology, 64*(1), 21–47. https://doi.org/10.1146/annurev-psych-113011-143739

[28] Sviženská, I. H., Dubový, P., & Šulcová, A. (2008). "Cannabinoid receptors 1 and 2 (CB1 and CB2), their distribution, ligands and functional involvement in nervous system structures — A short review." *Pharmacology, Biochemistry and Behavior, 90*(4), 501–511. https://doi.org/10.1016/j.pbb.2008.05.010

[29] Wright, K. L., Duncan, M., & Sharkey, K. A. (2008). "Cannabinoid CB2 receptors in the gastrointestinal tract: a regulatory system in states of inflammation." *British Journal of Pharmacology, 153*(2), 263–270. https://doi.org/10.1038/sj.bjp.0707486

[30] Castillo, P. E., Younts, T. J., Chávez, A. E., & Hashimotodani, Y. (2012). "Endocannabinoid signaling and synaptic function." *Neuron, 76*(1), 70–81. https://doi.org/10.1016/j.neuron.2012.09.020

[31] *Introduction to the Endocannabinoid System - NORML*. (2020, June 29). NORML. http://norml.org/library/item/introduction-to-the-endocannabinoid-system/

[32] Melamede, R. (2010). "Endocannabinoids: Multi-scaled, Global Homeostatic Regulators of Cells and Society." In: Minai, A., Braha, D., Bar-Yam, Y. (eds) Unifying Themes in Complex Systems. Springer, Berlin, Heidelberg. https://doi.org/10.1007/978-3-540-85081-6_28

[33] Di Marzo, V., Melck, D., Bisogno, T., & De Petrocellis, L. (1998). "Endocannabinoids: endogenous cannabinoid receptor ligands with neuromodulatory action." *Trends in Neurosciences, 21*(12), 521–528. https://doi.org/10.1016/s0166-2236(98)01283-1

The Effects of Cannabis

Brain & Nervous System	Modulates the neurotransmission rate via retrograde inhibition; Critical for homeostasis; Reduces gastrointestinal motility via the vagus nerve.
Nose	Increases sensitivity to odor and increases foraging behavior.
Mouth/Oral Cavity	Increases neural response to sweet taste; Regulation of taste sensitivity.
Gastrointestinal Tract	Increases preference and intake and affects the speed of peristalsis (movement in the intestinal tract).
Pancreas	Increases insulin secretion; Increases apoptotic activity and cancer cell death by increasing ceramide in cancer cells.
Liver	Increases lipogenesis and decreases insulin clearance.
Skeletal Muscle	Decreases insulin-dependent glucose uptake and decreases inflammation.
Adipose Tissue	Increases adipogenesis; Increases glucose uptake; Decreases oxidation of fatty acids; Decreases mitochondrial biogenesis and is a repository for THC.

A Primer 23

ECS & the Central Nervous System

The human brain is composed of distinct parts, such as the neocortex, the midbrain, and the limbic system.[34] From primitive life forms to humans, all mammals have the midbrain, the oldest part of the human brain. The midbrain is part of the brainstem that controls basic functions for life, such as heart rate and breathing. The limbic system is associated with emotional responses such as fear or fight-or-flight responses but also with memory or other complex behaviors such as feeding. The neocortex is the home of rational thinking and executive functions; this region is intensely connected with the previous ones.

Parts of the Brain Affected by Cannabis

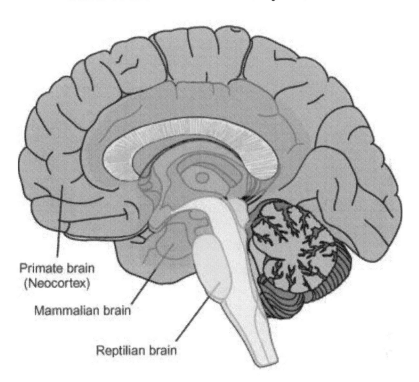

SOURCE: *Bernard J. Baars, Nicole M. Gage, in Cognition, Brain, and Consciousness (Second Edition), 2010*

---

[34] Baars BJ, Gage NM, editors. *Introduction to Cognitive Neuroscience*. 2nd ed. Elsevier: 2010. p. 421-442.

Reptilian Brain, or Midbrain	The oldest part of the brain. Critical for survival (fight-or-flight) instincts and reproductive functions. It perceives everything as black and white, life or death.
Cerebral Cortex	Evolutionarily the newest part of the brain. It plays a role in memory, thinking, perceptual awareness, and consciousness.
Limbic System	Responsible for emotion, feeling, and empathy.
Hypothalamus	Governs metabolic processes.
Hippocampus	Central to memory storage and retrieval.
Cerebellum	Governs muscle coordination and control.
Brain Stem	Controls many basic functions, including arousal, gag reflex, blood pressure, heart rate, and breathing. (NOTE: Cannabis has little or no effect on the brain stem because it contains little or no CB1 receptors).

The elements that make up the ECS are widely expressed in the human brain. Cannabinoid receptors and their ligands are found in the brain of all mammals, and are located throughout the central and peripheral nervous systems. CB1 receptors are located in the midbrain, hippocampus, cerebral cortex, and amygdala; the CB2 receptor, on the other hand, was considered exclusively peripheral for many years, but it is currently known to have central expression.[35]

In the brain, neurons communicate through specialized structures located as gaps between these cells, called synapses. At synapses, electrical signals between neurons are translated chemically through neurotransmitters such as dopamine, serotonin, or glutamate. These neurotransmitters are released by the presynaptic neuron and act on specific receptors. One of the main functions of the ECS is to modulate the communication between neurons by regulating, among other mechanisms, the release of **neurotransmitters**. For this, it acts retrogradely: the two main endocannabinoids, AEA and 2-AG, are synthesized on demand by the postsynaptic neuron and act predominantly by activating presynaptic cannabinoid receptors, leading to the inhibition of the release of several neurotransmitters.[36,37]

CB1 receptors are inhibitory G protein-coupled receptors (GPCRs) and are abundantly present in neurons, modulating neurotransmission.[38] In the brain, CB1 is found in greater density in regions such as the basal ganglia, substantia nigra, cerebellum, and hippocampus.[39,40,41] Such location facilitates its inhibitory action on the release of neurotransmitters and, when active, leads to a reduction in the accumulation of cyclic adenosine 3',5'-monophosphate (cAMP) and, consequently, to the inhibition of cAMP-dependent protein kinase (PKA). CB1 receptors can activate mitogen-activated protein kinases (MAPKs), involved in processes of cell migration

---

[35] Kendall, D. A., & Yudowski, G. A. (2017). "Cannabinoid receptors in the central nervous system: their signaling and roles in disease." *Frontiers in Cellular Neuroscience, 10.* https://doi.org/10.3389/fncel.2016.00294

[36] Mechoulam, R., & Parker, L. A. (2013). "The endocannabinoid system and the brain." *Annual Review of Psychology, 64*(1), 21–47. https://doi.org/10.1146/annurev-psych-113011-143739

[37] Di Marzo, V., Melck, D., Bisogno, T., & De Petrocellis, L. (1998). "Endocannabinoids: endogenous cannabinoid receptor ligands with neuromodulatory action." *Trends in Neurosciences, 21*(12), 521–528. https://doi.org/10.1016/s0166-2236(98)01283-1

[38] Piomelli, D. (2003). "The molecular logic of endocannabinoid signalling." *Nature Reviews Neuroscience, 4*(11), 873–884. https://doi.org/10.1038/nrn1247

[39] Mechoulam, R., & Parker, L. A. (2013). "The endocannabinoid system and the brain." *Annual Review of Psychology, 64*(1), 21–47. https://doi.org/10.1146/annurev-psych-113011-143739

[40] De Fonseca, F. R., Del Arco, I., Bermúdez-Silva, F. J., Bilbao, A., Cippitelli, A., & Navarro, M. (2004). "The Endocannabinoid System: Physiology and Pharmacology." *Alcohol and Alcoholism, 40*(1), 2–14. https://doi.org/10.1093/alcalc/agh110

[41] Demuth, D., & Molleman, A. (2006). "Cannabinoid signalling." *Life Sciences, 78*(6), 549–563. https://doi.org/10.1016/j.lfs.2005.05.055

and neuronal growth, representing one of the mechanisms by which endocannabinoids favor synaptic plasticity.[42] Another important factor involved in the activation of CB1 is that this receptor, as it is coupled to the G protein, is linked to several Ca2+ and K+ channels.[43] CB2 receptors, in turn, are located in microglia and neurons, but in lower concentrations than CB1 receptors.[44]

Several psychiatric and neurological disorders involve neurotransmission changes or neuronal excitability, such as migraines, seizure disorders, or attention deficit hyperactivity disorder (ADHD),[45,46,47,48,49] which could explain the therapeutic potential of cannabis in these conditions. One of the most studied neurotransmission systems in the context of medicinal cannabis is dopaminergic neurotransmission. Dopamine and its transporter play an important role in ECS functionality. Cannabinoid receptors colocalize with dopaminergic receptors, suggesting that cannabinoids may affect dopaminergic neurotransmission.[50,51,52]

The brain also undergoes age-related changes in structure and function, which include shrinkage of its tissue and consequent decrease in its mass,

---

[42] Demuth, D., & Molleman, A. (2006). "Cannabinoid signalling." *Life Sciences*, *78*(6), 549–563. https://doi.org/10.1016/j.lfs.2005.05.055

[43] Howlett, A. C. (2002). "The cannabinoid receptors." *Prostaglandins & Other Lipid Mediators*, *68–69*, 619–631. https://doi.org/10.1016/s0090-6980(02)00060-6

[44] Ashton, J. C., Friberg, D., Darlington, C. L., & Smith, P. F. (2006). "Expression of the cannabinoid CB2 receptor in the rat cerebellum: An immunohistochemical study." *Neuroscience Letters*, *396*(2), 113–116. https://doi.org/10.1016/j.neulet.2005.11.038

[45] During, M. J., & Spencer, D. D. (1993). "Extracellular hippocampal glutamate and spontaneous seizure in the conscious human brain." *The Lancet*, *341*(8861), 1607–1610. https://doi.org/10.1016/0140-6736(93)90754-5

[46] Áfra, J. (2000). "Cortical excitability in migraine." *Journal of Headache and Pain*, *1*(2), 73–81. https://doi.org/10.1007/pl00012181

[47] Coppola, G., & Schoenen, J. (2011). "Cortical excitability in chronic migraine." *Current Pain and Headache Reports*, *16*(1), 93–100. https://doi.org/10.1007/s11916-011-0231-1

[48] Bonansco, C., & Fuenzalida, M. (2016). "Plasticity of hippocampal Excitatory-Inhibitory balance: missing the synaptic control in the epileptic brain." *Neural Plasticity*, *2016*, 1–13. https://doi.org/10.1155/2016/8607038

[49] Mehta, T., Monegro, A., Nene, Y., Fayyaz, M., & Bollu, P. C. (2019). "Neurobiology of ADHD: a review." *Current Developmental Disorders Reports*, *6*(4), 235–240. https://doi.org/10.1007/s40474-019-00182-w

[50] Fernández-Ruiz, J. (2009). "The endocannabinoid system as a target for the treatment of motor dysfunction." *British Journal of Pharmacology*, *156*(7), 1029–1040. https://doi.org/10.1111/j.1476-5381.2008.00088.x

[51] Fitzgerald, M. L., Shobin, E., & Pickel, V. M. (2012). "Cannabinoid modulation of the dopaminergic circuitry: Implications for limbic and striatal output." *Progress in Neuro-Psychopharmacology and Biological Psychiatry*, *38*(1), 21–29. https://doi.org/10.1016/j.pnpbp.2011.12.004

[52] Covey, D. P., Mateo, Y., Sulzer, D., Cheer, J. F., & Lovinger, D. M. (2017). "Endocannabinoid modulation of dopamine neurotransmission." *Neuropharmacology*, *124*, 52–61. https://doi.org/10.1016/j.neuropharm.2017.04.033

loss of neuronal populations and increase in glial cells, decreased ability to produce new neurons, change in neurotransmission systems, decrease in cognitive function (in a variety of domains), decrease in motor speed and strength, and decrease in reaction time. Just as the brain and its cellular constituents change with age, so does the ECS,[53] which raises the possibility of modulating this system to prevent some of the deleterious effects derived from the aging process.

ECS & Mitochondria

The **mitochondria** are intracellular organelles present in all cells of all multicellular organisms except mammalian red blood cells.[54] One of the main functions of mitochondria is to convert high-energy molecules (such as lipids and amino acids) into **adenosine triphosphate (ATP)**, to be used as an energy source for cellular processes crucial for maintaining life.[55] "Originally, mitochondria were not an organelle but were separate from other cells," writes Martin Lee, author of *Smoke Signals: A Social History of Marijuana - Medical, Recreational, and Scientific* (2012). Lee postulates that about one and a half billion to two billion years ago, "...a cell swallowed an evolutionary precursor of a mitochondria. But instead of digesting it, the two living entities formed a symbiotic relationship. The host cell would provide nutrients and a safe place for the mitochondria to exist, and the mitochondria would carry out the [oxidative] process of cellular respiration, giving the host a more usable form of energy."

This symbiotic relationship had an important impact on multicellular organisms' emergence.[56]

---

[53] Bilkei-Gorzó, A. (2012). "The endocannabinoid system in normal and pathological brain aging." *Philosophical Transactions of the Royal Society B*, 367(1607), 3326–3341. https://doi.org/10.1098/rstb.2011.0388

[54] Zhang, Z., Cheng, J., Xu, F., Chen, Y., Du, J., Yuan, M., Feng, Z., Xu, X., & Yuan, S. (2011). "Red blood cell extrudes nucleus and mitochondria against oxidative stress." *IUBMB Life*, 63(7), 560–565. https://doi.org/10.1002/iub.490

[55] Dunn, J. (2023, February 13). *Physiology, adenosine triphosphate*. StatPearls - NCBI Bookshelf. https://www.ncbi.nlm.nih.gov/books/NBK553175/

[56] Noel. (2023, March 29). "Mitochondria Mysteries | Project CBD." *Project CBD*. https://projectcbd.org/science/mitochondria-mysteries/

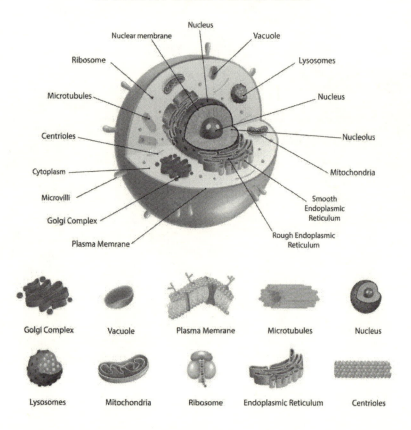

Cannabinoid receptors, in addition to their expression in the cell's plasma membrane, can also be found in the mitochondria.[57] It is estimated that 15% of all CB1 receptors are expressed in the mitochondrial membrane and muscle tissue, and about half of CB1 receptors are located in mitochondria.[58] Despite being found in different structures, CB1 receptors do not show structural differences. However, the effect of its activation can be quite

---

[57] Busquets-Garcia, A., Bains, J. S., & Marsicano, G. (2017). "CB1 Receptor Signaling in the Brain: Extracting Specificity from Ubiquity." *Neuropsychopharmacology*, 43(1), 4–20. https://doi.org/10.1038/npp.2017.206

[58] Mendizabal-Zubiaga, J., Melser, S., Bénard, G., Ramos, A., Reguero, L., Arrabal, S., Elezgarai, I., Gerrikagoitia, I., Suárez, J., De Fonseca, F. R., Puente, N., Marsicano, G., & Grandes, P. (2016). "Cannabinoid CB1 receptors are localized in striated muscle mitochondria and regulate mitochondrial respiration." *Frontiers in Physiology*, 7. https://doi.org/10.3389/fphys.2016.00476

different.[59,60,61] Associate researcher and science writer Adrian Devitt-Lee explains this difference:

> *Light switches may look the same from room to room, but they are connected to different circuits throughout the house, so turning the switch on or off in different places causes different results.*[62]

Examining the role of mitochondria can help shed light on the perplexing and confusing aspects sometimes associated with the ECS. Cannabinoid activity in mitochondria is complex. Under low-stress conditions, cannabinoids generally increase mitochondrial activity and cellular respiration, triggering a process called autophagic cell repair. Cannabinoids may also attenuate high-stress conditions and protect cells by decreasing mitochondrial activity.[63,64,65] The human body requires energy, and it obtains it in the form of adenosine triphosphate (ATP). ATP is produced in the mitochondria, but the creation of this energy source generates free radicals that can cause cell damage.[66,67] ECS modulation can reduce these effects by reducing free radicals.[68] This mechanism of action is even one of the attributes of the cannabis plant that is believed to contribute to its anti-inflammatory effect. Devitt-Lee explains further:

---

[59] *Involvement of Gi in the inhibition of adenylate cyclase by cannabimimetic drugs.* (1986, March 1). PubMed. https://pubmed.ncbi.nlm.nih.gov/2869405/

[60] Lauckner, J. E., Hille, B., & Mackie, K. (2005). "The cannabinoid agonist WIN55,212-2 increases intracellular calcium via CB_1 receptor coupling to $G_{q/11}$ G proteins." *Proceedings of the National Academy of Sciences of the United States of America, 102*(52), 19144–19149. https://doi.org/10.1073/pnas.0509588102

[61] Felder, C. C., & Glass, M. (1998). "cannabinoid Receptors And Their Endogenous Agonists." *Annual Review of Pharmacology and Toxicology, 38*(1), 179–200. https://doi.org/10.1146/annurev.pharmtox.38.1.179

[62] Noel. (2023, March 29). "Mitochondria Mysteries | Project CBD." *Project CBD.* https://projectcbd.org/science/mitochondria-mysteries/

[63] Codogno, P., & Meijer, A. J. (2005). "Autophagy and signaling: their role in cell survival and cell death." *Cell Death & Differentiation, 12*(S2), 1509–1518. https://doi.org/10.1038/sj.cdd.4401751

[64] Salazar, M., Carracedo, A., Salanueva, Í. J., Hernández-Tiedra, S., Lorente, M., Egia, A., Vázquez, P., Blázquez, C., Torres, S., García, S., Nowak, J. A., Fimia, G. M., Piacentini, M., Cecconi, F., Pandolfi, P. P., González-Feria, L., Iovanna, J., Guzmán, M., Boya, P., & Velasco, G. (2009). "Cannabinoid action induces autophagy-mediated cell death through stimulation of ER stress in human glioma cells." *Journal of Clinical Investigation, 119*(5), 1359–1372. https://doi.org/10.1172/jci37948

[65] Lee, X. C., Werner, E., & Falasca, M. (2021). "Molecular mechanism of autophagy and its regulation by cannabinoids in cancer." *Cancers, 13*(6), 1211. https://doi.org/10.3390/cancers13061211

[66] Murphy, M. P. (2008). "How mitochondria produce reactive oxygen species." *Biochemical Journal, 417*(1), 1–13. https://doi.org/10.1042/bj20081386

[67] Van Hameren, G., Campbell, G., Deck, M., Berthelot, J., Gautier, B., Quintana, P., Chrast, R., & Tricaud, N. (2019). "In vivo real-time dynamics of ATP and ROS production in axonal mitochondria show decoupling in mouse models of peripheral neuropathies." *Acta Neuropathologica Communications, 7*(1). https://doi.org/10.1186/s40478-019-0740-4

[68] Lipina, C., & Hundal, H. S. (2016). "Modulation of cellular redox homeostasis by the endocannabinoid system." *Open Biology, 6*(4), 150276. https://doi.org/10.1098/rsob.150276

> *Imagine trying to start a car simply by lighting a fuel tank. That's a lot of energy. A cell cannot handle the microscopic equivalent of an explosion, so the cell must use subtlety to harness that energy... Although mitochondria allow energy to be accessed at a relatively small amount rate, the process of cellular respiration (by which cells extract energy from nutrients) can still be harmful. The high-energy electrons discharge their energy in a multitude of complicated steps until the low-energy electron is finally released in an oxygen molecule.*[69]

Homeostasis

Homeostasis is the state of internal balance, physical and chemical, of physiological systems' maintenance. It is defined as "the tendency toward a relatively stable balance between interdependent elements, especially with the maintenance of physiological processes."[70] The ECS plays an important role in homeostasis and helps regulate essential functions such as pain, mood, digestion, sleep, and appetite, among others.[71,72]

Dr. Robert Meladmede, a retired biology professor at the University of Colorado, has written extensively on the effect of cannabinoids and cannabis on homeostasis. He claims:

> *Endocannabinoids are believed to have their evolutionary origin 600 million years ago. In the last [three decades] since the identification of cannabinoid receptors, research on the Endocannabinoid System has grown exponentially. (...) [Endocannabinoids] serve as modulators fundamental to energy homeostasis in many multicellular organisms, including all vertebrates. They have widespread biological activities that can often be attributed to their ability to minimize the negative consequences of free radicals."*[73]

---

[69] Noel. (2023, March 29). "Mitochondria Mysteries | Project CBD." *Project CBD.* https://projectcbd.org/science/mitochondria-mysteries/

[70] *Oxford Languages | The Home of Language Data.* (2022, August 26). https://en.oxforddictionaries.com/definition/homeostasis/

[71] Ligresti, A., Petrosino, S., & Di Marzo, V. (2009). "From endocannabinoid profiling to "endocannabinoid therapeutics." *Current Opinion in Chemical Biology, 13*(3), 321–331. https://doi.org/10.1016/j.cbpa.2009.04.615

[72] Battista, N., Di Tommaso, M., Bari, M., & Maccarrone, M. (2012). "The endocannabinoid system: an overview." *Frontiers in Behavioral Neuroscience, 6.* https://doi.org/10.3389/fnbeh.2012.00009

[73] Melamede, R. (2010). "Endocannabinoids: Multi-scaled, Global Homeostatic Regulators of Cells and Society." In: Minai, A., Braha, D., Bar-Yam, Y. (eds) *Unifying Themes in Complex Systems.* Springer, Berlin, Heidelberg. https://doi.org/10.1007/978-3-540-85081-6_28

Phytocannabinoids

Phytocannabinoids are plant-sourced cannabinoids that interact with the ECS. The binding between phytocannabinoids and key ECS receptors can be orthosteric or allosteric. The THC molecule binds to CB1 receptors and sends a signal into the cell.[74,75] This type of receptor binding is called orthosteric binding. Cannabidiol (CBD) binds allosterically to CB1, changing the conformation of the receptor to make it easier or more difficult for an orthosteric ligand to "fit" the receptor and activate or block it.[76,77] CBD can decrease THC-mediated euphoria when both are bound to CB1.[78] Furthermore, CBD also exhibits various therapeutic effects, including appetite stimulation, mood elevation, pain reduction, analgesia, and anti-inflammatory effects.[79] According to Dr. Deborah Malka, an allopathic physician and herbalist, when the dose of CBD exceeds the dose of THC, the CBD can not only interfere with the euphoric effects of the THC but also decrease the analgesic effect of the cannabis. CBD works to reduce pain more indirectly than THC by reducing inflammation.[80]

There are also structures, other than CB1 and CB2 receptors, that play a role in the effects of cannabis in the body. For example, CBD does not directly activate mitochondrial CB1 receptors. Instead, the CBD molecule binds to different receptors, including the sodium-calcium exchanger (NCX), found

---

[74] Russo, E. B. (2011). "Taming THC: potential cannabis synergy and phytocannabinoid-terpenoid entourage effects." *British Journal of Pharmacology, 163*(7), 1344–1364. https://doi.org/10.1111/j.1476-5381.2011.01238.x

[75] Russo, E. B., & Marcu, J. P. (2017b). "Cannabis Pharmacology: the usual suspects and a few promising leads." In *Advances in pharmacology* (pp. 67–134). https://doi.org/10.1016/bs.apha.2017.03.004

[76] Russo, E. B., & Marcu, J. P. (2017). Cannabis Pharmacology: the usual suspects and a few promising leads. In *Advances in pharmacology* (pp. 67–134). https://doi.org/10.1016/bs.apha.2017.03.004

[77] Thomas, A., Baillie, G., Phillips, A. M., Razdan, R. K., Ross, R. A., & Pertwee, R. G. (2007). "Cannabidiol displays unexpectedly high potency as an antagonist of CB$_1$and CB$_2$receptor agonists" *in vitro*. British Journal of Pharmacology, 150(5), 613–623. https://doi.org/10.1038/sj.bjp.0707133

[78] Dunn, J. (2023, February 13). *Physiology, adenosine triphosphate*. StatPearls - NCBI Bookshelf. https://www.ncbi.nlm.nih.gov/books/NBK553175/

[79] Russo, E. B., & Marcu, J. P. (2017a). "Cannabis Pharmacology: the usual suspects and a few promising leads." In *Advances in pharmacology* (pp. 67–134). https://doi.org/10.1016/bs.apha.2017.03.004

[80] Malka, D. (2021). *Medicinal cannabis: Pearls for Clinical Practice*. CRC Press.

on the surface of mitochondria.[81] Binding to NCX opens an ion channel to CB2 receptors, which in turn activates these receptors.[82]

CBD plays a role in the intracellular regulation of calcium levels. Different levels of calcium ions exert different effects. Under conditions of low cellular stress, characterized by low intracellular calcium around the mitochondria, CBD will increase stress by allowing calcium to flow out of the mitochondria. In contrast, under conditions of heightened stress, characterized by high intracellular calcium levels, CBD will do the exact opposite, allowing calcium to flow from the outside into the mitochondria (where calcium is stored) by opening the NCX. This bidirectional flow of calcium is regulated by NCX and is one of the mechanisms by which CBD facilitates cellular homeostasis and neuroprotection.[83]

The ECS is very robust and regulates several physiological as well as pathological processes. Cannabinoids, via the ECS, modulate neuronal activity and regulate the immune system. Many pathologies respond to exogenous cannabinoids, leading researchers to theorize that people with inflammatory conditions and/or conditions related to rapid neural transmission may be below the fifth percentile in terms of body production of one or more endogenous ECS constituents, the so-called ECS deficiency syndrome.[84] While this is just a theory, it could explain why cannabis and cannabinoids are beneficial for treating a wide spectrum of ailments.

Dr. Daniele Piomelli, a pharmacology professor at the University of California at Irvine, postulates that many patients suffering from ADHD, bipolar disorder, panic attacks, and Tourette's Syndrome may have an

---

[81] Ryan, D., Drysdale, A. J., Lafourcade, C., Pertwee, R. G., & Platt, B. (2009). "Cannabidiol Targets Mitochondria to Regulate Intracellular Ca^{2+} Levels." *The Journal of Neuroscience, 29*(7), 2053–2063. https://doi.org/10.1523/jneurosci.4212-08.2009

[82] Maslov, L. N., Khaliulin, I., Zhang, Y., Крылатов, A. B., Naryzhnaya, N. V., Mechoulam, R., De Petrocellis, L., & Downey, J. M. (2015). "Prospects for creation of cardioprotective drugs based on cannabinoid receptor agonists." *Journal of Cardiovascular Pharmacology and Therapeutics, 21*(3), 262–272. https://doi.org/10.1177/1074248415612593

[83] Chan, J. Z., & Duncan, R. E. (2021). "Regulatory effects of cannabidiol on mitochondrial functions: a review." *Cells, 10*(5), 1251. https://doi.org/10.3390/cells10051251

[84] *Clinical endocannabinoid deficiency (CECD): can this concept explain therapeutic benefits of cannabis in migraine, fibromyalgia, irritable bowel syndrome and other treatment-resistant conditions?* (2004, April 1). PubMed. https://pubmed.ncbi.nlm.nih.gov/15159679/

endocannabinoid deficiency.[85] Interestingly, these conditions are related to excessive speed and frequency of neurotransmission.[86,87,88]

---

[85] Beltramo, M., De Fonseca, F. R., Navarro, M., Calignano, A., Gorriti, M. Á., Grammatikopoulos, G., Sadile, A. G., Giuffrida, A., & Piomelli, D. (2000). "Reversal of Dopamine D₂Receptor Responses by an Anandamide Transport Inhibitor." *The Journal of Neuroscience*, 20(9), 3401–3407. https://doi.org/10.1523/jneurosci.20-09-03401.2000

[86] Coplan, J. D., & Lydiard, R. B. (1998). Brain circuits in panic disorder. *Biological Psychiatry*, 44(12), 1264–1276. https://doi.org/10.1016/s0006-3223(98)00300-x

[87] Manji, H. K. (2003, October 1). *The underlying neurobiology of bipolar disorder*. PubMed Central (PMC). https://www.ncbi.nlm.nih.gov/pmc/articles/PMC1525098/

[88] Felling, R. J., & Singer, H. S. (2011). "Neurobiology of Tourette Syndrome: Current status and need for further investigation: Table 1." *The Journal of Neuroscience*, 31(35), 12387–12395. https://doi.org/10.1523/jneurosci.0150-11.2011

Constituents & Chemical Characteristics of Cannabis

The understanding of the basic chemistry of cannabis began with T. & H. Smith in 1846 when they stated that cannabis resin had soporific, calming, anxiolytic, and other properties.[89] MJ Personne closely followed the Smiths' findings in 1857, claiming that the activity of the drug depended on its volatile oil.[90] At the time, it was known that cannabis vapor could be intoxicating. Personne was able to split the oil into two parts—a fluid known as cannabene ($C_{18}H_{20}$) and a crystallized solid known as cannabene hydride ($C_{18}H_{22}$).

There was an over 100-year gap between this research and the characterization of the plant's active chemical constituents. The molecular structure of Δ^9-tetrahydrocannabinol (THC) was first isolated and identified in 1964 by Israeli scientists Raphael Mechoulam and Yehiel Gaoni.[91] THC is the most euphoric of the phytocannabinoids and, along with CBD, one of the most abundant plant constituents.[92] One of the first modern studies involving a cannabinoid was carried out in 1949 by H.H. Ramsey and J.P. Davis, who found that synthetic THC was useful for treating intractable epilepsy.[93] The first known formal modern physiological research on cannabis was done at Harvard in 1968 by Dr. Andrew Weil.[94] Along with these studies, there have been many double-blind human studies of the medicinal application of cannabis carried out in the first decade of the twenty-first century by GW Pharmaceuticals in the United Kingdom and the Center for Medicinal Cannabis Research (CMCR) based at the University of California, San Diego, School of Medicine.

---

[89] Dixon, W. E. (1899, November 11). *The Pharmacology of Cannabis Indica*. PubMed Central (PMC). https://www.ncbi.nlm.nih.gov/pmc/articles/PMC2412674/

[90] Personne MJ. "Rapport sur le concours relative d l'analyse du chanure, présenté au nom de la Société de Pharmacie." *Journal de Pharmacie et de Chimie*. 1857;31.

[91] Gaoni, Y., & Mechoulam, R. (1964). "Isolation, structure, and partial synthesis of an active constituent of hashish". *Journal of the American Chemical Society*, 86(8), 1646–1647. https://doi.org/10.1021/ja01062a046

[92] Maayah, Z. H., Takahara, S., Ferdaoussi, M., & Dyck, J. R. (2020). "The molecular mechanisms that underpin the biological benefits of full-spectrum cannabis extract in the treatment of neuropathic pain and inflammation." *Biochimica Et Biophysica Acta (BBA) - Molecular Basis of Disease*, 1866(7), 165771. https://doi.org/10.1016/j.bbadis.2020.165771

[93] Davis JP, Ramsey HH. "Antiepileptic action of marihuana active substances." In Fed. Proc. 1949;8:284-5.

[94] Weil A. *The Natural Mind: An Investigation of Drugs and the Higher Consciousness*. Houghton Mifflin Harcourt, 1972.

Cannabis contains at least 512 different molecules, including flavonoids, terpenes, and phytocannabinoids:[95]

- Phytocannabinoids are 21-carbon molecules that act on CB1 or CB2 receptors. The main euphorigenic substance belonging to this group is THC. At least 113–150 other phytocannabinoids synthesized by the plant have been identified. These include, in addition to THC and CBD, other molecules such as cannabinol (CBN), cannabigerol (CBG), and cannabichromene (CBC).[96,97]
- Terpenes are the molecules that contribute to cannabis cultivars' distinctive odors.[98]
- **Flavonoids** are color pigments and antioxidants found in fruits, vegetables, and herbs, including cannabis.[99]

Cannabis plant matter also contains chlorophyll, green resin, albumin, lignin, sugars, and salts such as potassium nitrate, silica, and phosphates, among other molecules.[100]

---

[95] Aizpurua-Olaizola, O., Soydaner, U., Öztürk, E., Schibano, D., Simsir, Y., Navarro, P., Etxebarría, N., & Usobiaga, A. (2016). "Evolution of the Cannabinoid and Terpene Content during the Growth of *Cannabis sativa* Plants from Different Chemotypes." *Journal of Natural Products*, 79(2), 324–331. https://doi.org/10.1021/acs.jnatprod.5b00949

[96] Russo, E. B., & Marcu, J. P. (2017a). "Cannabis Pharmacology: the usual suspects and a few promising leads." In *Advances in pharmacology* (pp. 67–134). https://doi.org/10.1016/bs.apha.2017.03.004

[97] Sampson, P. B. (2020). "Phytocannabinoid Pharmacology: Medicinal Properties of *Cannabis sativa* Constituents Aside from the 'Big Two.'" *Journal of Natural Products*, 84(1), 142–160. https://doi.org/10.1021/acs.jnatprod.0c00965

[98] Sommano, S. R., Chittasupho, C., Ruksiriwanich, W., & Jantrawut, P. (2020). "The cannabis terpenes." *Molecules*, 25(24), 5792. https://doi.org/10.3390/molecules25245792

[99] Bautista, J. L., Song, Y., & Tian, L. (2021). "Flavonoids in *Cannabis sativa*: Biosynthesis, Bioactivities, and Biotechnology." *ACS Omega*, 6(8), 5119–5123. https://doi.org/10.1021/acsomega.1c00318

[100] Turner, C. E., ElSohly, M. A., & Boeren, E. G. (1980). "Constituents of Cannabis sativa L. XVII. A Review of the Natural Constituents." *Journal of Natural Products*, 43(2), 169–234. https://doi.org/10.1021/np50008a001

Chemical Constituents of Cannabis

Constituent	Number
Aldehydes	13
Amino acids	18
Elements	9
Enzymes	2
Fatty acids	22
Flavonoids	21
Glycoproteins	6
Hydrocarbons	50
Ketones	13
Lactones	1
Nitrogen compounds	27
Non-cannabinoid phenols	25
Pigments	2
Proteins	3
Simple acids	21
Simple alcohols	7
Simple esters	12
Steroids	11
Sugars and related compounds	34
Terpenes	200
Vitamins	1

Cannabinoid Conversions

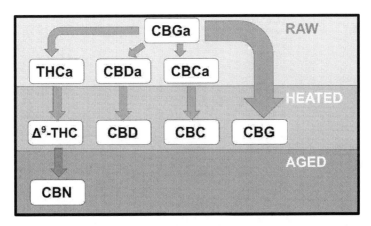

All cannabinoids biosynthesize first as CBGa before converting to THCa, CBDa, or CBCa, depending on both plant genetics and environmental conditions. As these compounds age and degrade or are heated they decarboxylate, or lose a carboxyl group, and convert to their active counterparts, THC, CBD, and CBG. As THC ages, it degrades into CBN.

Therapeutic Potential of Phytocannabinoids

Although THC is considered the pharmacologically psychoactive constituent of cannabis and, consequently, the most studied, other phytocannabinoids such as CBD, CBN, and CBG have attracted a lot of attention for their therapeutic application.

Cannabigerol (CBG)

CBG is the "mother cannabinoid." It is the precursor to all other cannabinoids and is converted into THCa, CBDa, and CBCa as the plant matures. CBG has anticancer and anti-inflammatory properties and slows down bacterial growth.[101,102,103]

---

[101] Russo, E. B., & Marcu, J. P. (2017a). "Cannabis Pharmacology: the usual suspects and a few promising leads." In *Advances in pharmacology* (pp. 67–134). https://doi.org/10.1016/bs.apha.2017.03.004

[102] Sampson, P. B. (2020). "Phytocannabinoid Pharmacology: Medicinal Properties of *Cannabis sativa* Constituents Aside from the 'Big Two.'" *Journal of Natural Products*, *84*(1), 142–160. https://doi.org/10.1021/acs.jnatprod.0c00965

[103] Nachnani, R., Raup-Konsavage, W. M., & Vrana, K. E. (2020). "The pharmacological case for cannabigerol." *Journal of Pharmacology and Experimental Therapeutics*, *376*(2), 204–212. https://doi.org/10.1124/jpet.120.000340

Cannabichromene (CBC)

First discovered in 1966, CBC has not been as widely studied;[104] there are no more than 75 articles published on PubMed that make specific references to CBC. Based on the research available, it is believed that CBC can act as an analgesic, sleep aid, antispasmodic, anti-inflammatory, antimicrobial, antifungal, anticancer agent, and bone growth promoter.[105,106,107] Freshly harvested dried cannabis contains significant amounts of CBC.[108]

Cannabinol (CBN)

First isolated in 1896, CBN is a byproduct of the degradation of THC.[109,110] CBN binds weakly to cannabinoid receptors.[111,112] There are over 500 papers published in scientific literature specific to CBN. Several articles document the therapeutic potential of CBN, which includes its ability to induce sleep, alleviate pain and spasticity, delay symptoms of Lou Gehrig's disease, increase appetite, and prevent the spread of certain antibiotic-resistant

---

[104] Mechoulam, R., Yagnitinsky, B., & Gaoni, Y. (1968). "Hashish. XII. Stereoelectronic factor in the chloranil dehydrogenation of cannabinoids. Total synthesis of dl-cannabichromene." *Journal of the American Chemical Society, 90*(9), 2418–2420. https://doi.org/10.1021/ja01011a037

[105] Wirth, P. W., Watson, E., ElSohly, M. A., Turner, C. E., & Murphy, J. C. (1980). "Anti-inflammatory properties of cannabichromene." *Life Sciences, 26*(23), 1991–1995. https://doi.org/10.1016/0024-3205(80)90631-1

[106] Davis, W. S., & Hatoum, N. S. (1983). "Neurobehavioral actions of cannabichromene and interactions with Δ9-tetrahydrocannabinol." *General Pharmacology-the Vascular System, 14*(2), 247–252. https://doi.org/10.1016/0306-3623(83)90004-6

[107] Davis, W. S., & Hatoum, N. S. (1983b). Neurobehavioral actions of cannabichromene and interactions with Δ9-tetrahydrocannabinol. *General Pharmacology-the Vascular System, 14*(2), 247–252. https://doi.org/10.1016/0306-3623(83)90004-6

[108] Turner, C. E., & ElSohly, M. A. (1981). "Biological Activity of Cannabichromene, its Homologs and Isomers." *The Journal of Clinical Pharmacology, 21*(S1). https://doi.org/10.1002/j.1552-4604.1981.tb02606.x

[109] Turner, C. E., & ElSohly, M. A. (1979). "Constituents of *cannabis sativa*L. XVI. A possible decomposition pathway of Δ^9-tetrahydrocannabinol to cannabinol." *Journal of Heterocyclic Chemistry, 16*(8), 1667–1668. https://doi.org/10.1002/jhet.5570160834

[110] Russo, E. B., & Marcu, J. P. (2017a). "Cannabis Pharmacology: the usual suspects and a few promising leads." In *Advances in pharmacology* (pp. 67–134). https://doi.org/10.1016/bs.apha.2017.03.004

[111] Rhee, M. H., Vogel, Z., Barg, J., Bayewitch, M., Levy, R., Hanŭs, L., Breuer, A., & Mechoulam, R. (1997). "Cannabinol derivatives: binding to cannabinoid receptors and inhibition of adenylyl cyclase." *Journal of Medicinal Chemistry, 40*(20), 3228–3233. https://doi.org/10.1021/jm970126f

[112] Russo, E. B., & Marcu, J. P. (2017a). "Cannabis Pharmacology: the usual suspects and a few promising leads." In *Advances in pharmacology* (pp. 67–134). https://doi.org/10.1016/bs.apha.2017.03.004

pathogens such as Methicillin-resistant Staphylococcus aureus (MRSA).[113] Combining THC with CBN produces potentiated sedative effects.[114]

Tetrahydrocannabivarin (THCV)

The medicinal properties of THCV include appetite suppression and antiepileptic properties.[115,116] THCV is currently being researched as a treatment for metabolic disorders, including diabetes.[117]

Cannabidiol (CBD)

CBD was first identified in 1940, and its specific chemical structure was determined in 1963.[118] Many researchers believe that CBD has substantial therapeutic potential. Studies suggest a wide range of possible therapeutic effects of CBD in various conditions, including Alzheimer's disease, Parkinson's disease, nausea, cancer, cerebral ischemia, diabetes, rheumatoid arthritis, and other inflammatory diseases.[119] CBD acts as an analgesic, sleep aid, spasm reliever, and anxiety reducer. It also has anti-inflammatory potential, vasodilator, anticonvulsant, the ability to lower blood glucose levels, reduce contractions of the small intestine, promotes bone growth,

---

[113] *Ibid.*

[114] Karniol, I. G., Shirakawa, I., Takahashi, R. N., Knobel, E., & Musty, R. E. (1975). "Effects of &Delta9-Tetrahydrocannabinol and Cannabinol in Man." *Pharmacology, 13*(6), 502–512. https://doi.org/10.1159/000136944

[115] Abioye, A. O., Ayodele, O., Marinkovic, A., Patidar, R., Akinwekomi, A., & Sanyaolu, A. (2020). "Δ9-Tetrahydrocannabivarin (THCV): a commentary on potential therapeutic benefit for the management of obesity and diabetes." *Journal of Cannabis Research, 2*(1). https://doi.org/10.1186/s42238-020-0016-7

[116] Hill, A. J., Weston, S. E., Jones, N. A., Smith, I., Bevan, S., Williamson, E. M., Stephens, G. J., Williams, C., & Whalley, B. J. (2010). "Δ9-Tetrahydrocannabivarin suppresses in vitro epileptiform and in vivo seizure activity in adult rats." *Epilepsia, 51*(8), 1522–1532. https://doi.org/10.1111/j.1528-1167.2010.02523.x

[117] Abioye, A. O., Ayodele, O., Marinkovic, A., Patidar, R., Akinwekomi, A., & Sanyaolu, A. (2020). "Δ9-Tetrahydrocannabivarin (THCV): a commentary on potential therapeutic benefit for the management of obesity and diabetes." *Journal of Cannabis Research, 2*(1). https://doi.org/10.1186/s42238-020-0016-7

[118] Mechoulam, R., & Shvo, Y. (1963). "Hashish—I." *Tetrahedron, 19*(12), 2073–2078. https://doi.org/10.1016/0040-4020(63)85022-x

[119] Zuardi, A. W. (2008). "Cannabidiol: from an inactive cannabinoid to a drug with wide spectrum of action." *Revista Brasileira De Psiquiatria, 30*(3), 271–280. https://doi.org/10.1590/s1516-44462008000300015

slow growth bacterial, inhibits the growth of cancer cells, and is neuroprotective and antiemetic.[120,121,122]

CBD was believed to not affect CB1 or CB2 receptors. Indeed, CBD is able to modulate THC-induced symptoms by binding to an allosteric site of the CB1 receptor,[123] after THC binds to the orthosteric site. This mechanism seems to be responsible for the partial decrease in the euphoric effect of THC. Some studies claim that CBD also suppresses FAAH,[124] decreasing endocannabinoid degradation and potentiating its effects. A Reading School of Pharmacy (UK) team found that CBD has the potential to prevent seizures with few side effects, such as uncontrollable tremors, that accompany many commonly prescribed anti-epileptic drugs.[125] CBD has also worked as an adjunct to other pharmaceutical treatments to manage epilepsy.[126]

Cannabinoid Acids

The main phytocannabinoid components of raw cannabis come in the form of acids such as THCa, CBDa, CBGa, and CBCa, among others.[127] Preliminary research suggests that acidic cannabinoids possess most of the anti-inflammatory properties that cannabis has to offer, but more robust research is still needed.

---

[120] Russo, E. B., & Marcu, J. P. (2017a). "Cannabis Pharmacology: the usual suspects and a few promising leads." In *Advances in pharmacology* (pp. 67–134). https://doi.org/10.1016/bs.apha.2017.03.004

[121] Peng, J., Fan, M., An, C., Ni, F., Huang, W., & Luo, J. (2022). "A narrative review of molecular mechanism and therapeutic effect of cannabidiol (CBD)." *Basic & Clinical Pharmacology & Toxicology, 130*(4), 439–456. https://doi.org/10.1111/bcpt.13710

[122] Li, L., Jin, F., Sun, L., Xuan, Y., Li, W., Li, Y., Yang, S., Zhu, B., Tian, X., Li, S., Zhao, L., Dang, R., Jiao, T., Zhang, H., & Wen, N. (2022). "Cannabidiol Promotes Osteogenic Differentiation of Bone Marrow Mesenchymal Stem Cells in the Inflammatory Microenvironment via the CB2-dependent p38 MAPK Signaling Pathway." *International Journal of Stem Cells, 15*(4), 405–414. https://doi.org/10.15283/ijsc21152

[123] Thomas, A., Baillie, G., Phillips, A. M., Razdan, R. K., Ross, R. A., & Pertwee, R. G. (2007b). "Cannabidiol displays unexpectedly high potency as an antagonist of CB_1 and CB_2 receptor agonists *in vitro*." *British Journal of Pharmacology, 150*(5), 613–623. https://doi.org/10.1038/sj.bjp.0707133

[124] Product, A. F.-. H. O. (2016, October 24). *CBD vs NICOTINE*. Meet Harmony. https://meetharmony.com/2016/10/24/cbd-non-psychoactive/

[125] Jones, N. A., Hill, A. J., Smith, I., Bevan, S., Cm, W., Whalley, B. J., & Stephens, G. J. (2009). "Cannabidiol Displays Antiepileptiform and Antiseizure Properties In Vitro and In Vivo." *Journal of Pharmacology and Experimental Therapeutics, 332*(2), 569–577. https://doi.org/10.1124/jpet.109.159145

[126] Geffrey, A. L., Pollack, S. F., Bruno, P., & Thiele, E. A. (2015). "Drug-drug interaction between clobazam and cannabidiol in children with refractory epilepsy." *Epilepsia, 56*(8), 1246–1251. https://doi.org/10.1111/epi.13060

[127] Maayah, Z. H., Takahara, S., Ferdaoussi, M., & Dyck, J. R. (2020). "The molecular mechanisms that underpin the biological benefits of full-spectrum cannabis extract in the treatment of neuropathic pain and inflammation." *Biochimica Et Biophysica Acta (BBA) - Molecular Basis of Disease, 1866*(7), 165771. https://doi.org/10.1016/j.bbadis.2020.165771

Cannabinoids in the acid form undergo a chemical change called **decarboxylation**, i.e. removal of a carboxyl group, originating their related neutral compounds. This can happen over time with drying or with heat.[128] The acidic form of THC (THCa) does not cause euphoria. This is likely because the carboxyl group affects the way the THCa molecule crosses the blood-brain barrier.[129]

---

[128] *Ibid.*

[129] Russo, E. B., & Marcu, J. P. (2017a). "Cannabis Pharmacology: the usual suspects and a few promising leads." In *Advances in pharmacology* (pp. 67–134). https://doi.org/10.1016/bs.apha.2017.03.004

Therapeutic Potential of Cannabinoids

	THC	THCa	THCV	CBN	CBD	CBDa	CBC	CBCa	CBG	CBGa
Pain Relief	✓		✓	✓		✓	✓		✓	✓
Inflammation reduction		✓	✓	✓		✓	✓		✓	✓
Appetite suppression			✓			✓				
Appetite stimulation	✓					✓				
Vomiting and Nausea Reduction	✓					✓				
Reduced small bowel contractions						✓				
Anxiolytic						✓				
Tranquilizer/ psychosis maintenance						✓				
Seizure Reduction		✓	✓	✓		✓				
Suppression of muscle spasms	✓		✓	✓		✓				
Sleep inducing effect						✓				
Decreased effectiveness of the immune system						✓				
Reduction in blood sugar levels			✓	✓		✓				
Prevention of nervous system degeneration						✓				
Psoriasis treatment						✓				
Reduced risk of clogged arteries						✓				
Kills/decreases bacteria growth						✓	✓		✓	
Fungal infections treatment						✓	✓	✓	✓	
Inhibition of tumor growth		✓				✓	✓		✓	
Bone growth promotion			✓			✓		✓	✓	

Flavonoids

Flavonoids are pigments found in almost all fruits and vegetables. Not only are they powerful antioxidants, but they also have anti-inflammatory and immune-boosting benefits.[130]

One of the best-known flavonoids is quercetin, which is found in abundance in red onions, kale, cherries, broccoli, tea, and cannabis, among other plants. Quercetin is anti-inflammatory, may alleviate allergy symptoms, and lower blood pressure, among other effects.[131]

The flavonoids Cannflavin-A (CFL-A), Cannflavin-B (CFL-B), and Cannflavin-C (CFL-C) were first identified in cannabis, and initially, like cannabinoids thought to be unique to it, are now starting to be identified in other plants too.[132,133] More research is needed to understand the effects and botanical synergies of flavonoids.

Terpenes

Terpenes are present in all plants, with over 50,000 substances currently known in nature. These molecules can be classified by the number of repeating units of a 5-carbon molecule called isoprene. They are essential oils that exist as monoterpenes, diterpenes, or sesquiterpenes.[134] They are more volatile aromatic molecules than phytocannabinoids since their presence is more related to the freshness and temperature of cannabis. The fresher and colder the cannabis is, the better the preservation of the terpenes. More than 200 terpenes have been isolated from cannabis, and each cultivar contains a

---

[130] Bautista, J. L., Song, Y., & Tian, L. (2021b). "Flavonoids in *Cannabis sativa*: Biosynthesis, Bioactivities, and Biotechnology." *ACS Omega, 6*(8), 5119–5123. https://doi.org/10.1021/acsomega.1c00318

[131] David, A. V. A., Arulmoli, R., & Parasuraman, S. (2016). "Overviews of biological importance of quercetin: A bioactive flavonoid." *Pharmacognosy Reviews, 10*(20), 84. https://doi.org/10.4103/0973-7847.194044

[132] Rea, K. A., Casaretto, J. A., Al-Abdul-Wahid, M. S., Sukumaran, A., Geddes-McAlister, J., Rothstein, S. J., & Akhtar, T. A. (2019). "Biosynthesis of cannflavins A and B from Cannabis sativa L." *Phytochemistry, 164*, 162–171. https://doi.org/10.1016/j.phytochem.2019.05.009

[133] Abdel-Kader MS, Radwan MM, Metwaly AM, Eissa IH, Hazekamp A, Sohly MA. Chemistry and Biological Activities of Cannflavins of the Cannabis Plant. Cannabis Cannabinoid Res. 2023 Dec;8(6):974-985. doi: 10.1089/can.2023.0128. Epub 2023 Sep 27. Erratum in: Cannabis Cannabinoid Res. 2024 Jan 12;:. PMID: 37756221; PMCID: PMC10714118

[134] Ninkuu, V., Lin, Z., Yan, J., Fu, Z., Yang, T., & Zeng, H. (2021). "Biochemistry of terpenes and recent advances in plant protection." *International Journal of Molecular Sciences, 22*(11), 5710. https://doi.org/10.3390/ijms22115710

unique terpene profile that strongly influences its characteristic aroma and flavor.[135,136]

Terpenes also have therapeutic value and are found in many plants, such as citrus fruits, flowers, pepper, and other spices. For centuries, spices have been used therapeutically for their terpene profiles. Here are some examples of terpenes and their therapeutic applications.

Myrcene

Myrcene is abundant in hops and mangoes and acts as a sedative, hypnotic, and muscle relaxant.[137,138] It may also be used as an analgesic, anti-inflammatory, antipsychotic, antispasmodic, anti-anxiety (anxiolytic), antioxidant, and for its anticancer and anti-aging properties.[139,140,141]

α-pinene

Some texts say that α-pinene is the most common natural terpene. Its medical uses are due to its anti-inflammatory, gastroprotective,

---

[135] Sommano, S. R., Chittasupho, C., Ruksiriwanich, W., & Jantrawut, P. (2020). "The cannabis terpenes." *Molecules, 25*(24), 5792. https://doi.org/10.3390/molecules25245792

[136] Lawless J. *The Illustrated Encyclopedia of Essential Oils: The Complete Guide to the Use of Oils in Aromatherapy and Herbalism.* Element: Shaftesbury, Dorset; Rockport, MA. 1995. p. 256

[137] Vale, T. G. D., Furtado, E. C., Santos, J., & Viana, G. S. B. (2002). "Central effects of citral, myrcene and limonene, constituents of essential oil chemotypes from Lippia alba (Mill.) N.E. Brown." *Phytomedicine, 9*(8), 709–714. https://doi.org/10.1078/094471102321621304

[138] Bisset NG, Wichtl M. *Herbal Drugs and Phytopharmaceuticals: A Handbook for Practice on a Scientific Basis.* 3rd ed. Medpharm Scientific Publishers: Stuttgarr; CRC Press: Boca Raton. 2004. 704 p.

[139] Rao, V. S. N., Menezes, A. M. S., & Viana, G. S. B. (1990). "Effect of myrcene on nociception in mice." *Journal of Pharmacy and Pharmacology, 42*(12), 877–878. https://doi.org/10.1111/j.2042-7158.1990.tb07046.x

[140] De-Oliveira, A., Pinto, L. F. R., & Paumgartten, F. J. R. (1997). "In vitro inhibition of CYP2B1 monooxygenase by β-myrcene and other monoterpenoid compounds." *Toxicology Letters, 92*(1), 39–46. https://doi.org/10.1016/s0378-4274(97)00034-9

[141] Surendran, S., Qassadi, F., Surendran, G., Lilley, D., & Heinrich, M. (2021). "Myrcene—What are the potential health benefits of this flavouring and aroma agent?" *Frontiers in Nutrition, 8.* https://doi.org/10.3389/fnut.2021.699666

antibacterial, and **anxiolytic** potential.[142,143,144,145,146] α-pinene also acts as a bronchodilator and is an **acetylcholinesterase inhibitor** that may aid memory.[147,148] This terpene is associated with pine trees and turpentine and is probably one of the reasons why a walk in a pine forest can be so relaxing. Furthermore, α-pinene may limit some of THC's euphorigenic effects.[149,150]

Limonene

Limonene is often found in citrus fruits and has anxiolytic, antidepressant, gastroprotective, antimicrobial, and antispasmodic properties.[151,152,153,154]

---

[142] *Comparative study of different essential oils of Bupleurum gibraltaricum Lamarck.* (1989, April 1). PubMed. https://pubmed.ncbi.nlm.nih.gov/2772005/

[143] Raman, A., Weir, U., & Bloomfield, S. F. (1995). "Antimicrobial effects of tea-tree oil and its major components on Staphylococcus aureus, Staph. epidermidis and Propionibacterium acnes." *Letters in Applied Microbiology, 21*(4), 242–245. https://doi.org/10.1111/j.1472-765x.1995.tb01051.x

[144] Köse, E. O., Deniz, İ. G., Sarıkürkçü, C., Aktaş, Ö., & Yavuz, M. C. (2010). "Chemical composition, antimicrobial and antioxidant activities of the essential oils of Sideritis erythrantha Boiss. and Heldr. (var. erythrantha and var. cedretorum P.H. Davis) endemic in Turkey." *Food and Chemical Toxicology, 48*(10), 2960–2965. https://doi.org/10.1016/j.fct.2010.07.033

[145] Da Silva, A. C. R., Lopes, P. M., Azevedo, M. M. B., Costa, D. G., Alviano, C. S., & Alviano, D. S. (2012). "Biological activities of A-Pinene and B-Pinene enantiomers." *Molecules, 17*(6), 6305–6316. https://doi.org/10.3390/molecules17066305

[146] Kasuya, H., Okada, N., Kubohara, M., Satou, T., Masuo, Y., & Koike, K. (2014). "Expression of BDNF and TH mRNA in the brain following inhaled administration of A-Pinene." *Phytotherapy Research, 29*(1), 43–47. https://doi.org/10.1002/ptr.5224

[147] Falk, A., Hagberg, M., Löf, A., Wigaeus-Hjelm, E., & Wang, Z. P. (1990). "Uptake, distribution and elimination of alpha-pinene in man after exposure by inhalation." *Scandinavian Journal of Work, Environment & Health*, 16(5), 372–378. https://doi.org/10.5271/sjweh.1771

[148] Perry, N. S. L., Houghton, P. J., Theobald, A., Jenner, P., & Perry, E. K. (2000). "In-vitro Inhibition of Human Erythrocyte Acetylcholinesterase by *Salvia lavandulaefolia* Essential Oil and Constituent Terpenes." *Journal of Pharmacy and Pharmacology, 52*(7), 895–902. https://doi.org/10.1211/0022357001774598

[149] Russo, E. B. (2011). "Taming THC: potential cannabis synergy and phytocannabinoid-terpenoid entourage effects." *British Journal of Pharmacology, 163*(7), 1344–1364. https://doi.org/10.1111/j.1476-5381.2011.01238.x

[150] Russo, E. B., & Marcu, J. P. (2017a). "Cannabis Pharmacology: the usual suspects and a few promising leads". In *Advances in pharmacology* (pp. 67–134). https://doi.org/10.1016/bs.apha.2017.03.004

[151] Onawunmi, G. O., Yisak, W., & Ogunlana, E. O. (1984). "Antibacterial constituents in the essential oil of Cymbopogon citratus (DC.) Stapf." *Journal of Ethnopharmacology, 12*(3), pp. 279–286. https://doi.org/10.1016/0378-8741(84)90057-6

[152] Komori, T., Fujiwara, R., Tanida, M., Nomura, J., & Yokoyama, M. (1995). "Effects of citrus fragrance on immune function and depressive states." *Neuroimmunomodulation, 2*(3), 174–180. https://doi.org/10.1159/000096889

[153] Carvalho-Freitas, M., & Da Costa, M. K. M. (2002). "Anxiolytic and Sedative Effects of Extracts and Essential Oil from Citrus aurantium L." *Biological & Pharmaceutical Bulletin, 25*(12), 1629–1633. https://doi.org/10.1248/bpb.25.1629

[154] Harris B. "Phytotherapeutic uses of essential oils." In: *Handbook of essential oils: Science, technology, and applications*. CRC Press: Boca Raton. 2010. pp. 315-352.

Like α-pinene, limonene limits the euphorigenic effect of THC.[155] Limonene can be used to help prevent and treat cancer and has immunostimulatory properties.[156,157] Its anti-inflammatory properties aid in the treatment of autoimmune diseases and connective tissue disorders such as degenerative arthritis, bursitis, rheumatoid arthritis, systemic lupus, ankylosing spondylitis, and fibromyalgia.[158] It also helps kill tumor cells and aids in skin healing by promoting cell regeneration.[159,160]

Linalool

Linalool is found in a variety of flowers, most notably lavender, as well as mint, cinnamon, and some fungi. It also has anxiolytic, sedative, anticonvulsant, analgesic, antineoplastic, anesthetic, and antipsychotic properties.[161,162,163,164,165,166]

---

[155] Russo, E. B. (2011). "Taming THC: potential cannabis synergy and phytocannabinoid-terpenoid entourage effects." *British Journal of Pharmacology*, *163*(7), 1344–1364. https://doi.org/10.1111/j.1476-5381.2011.01238.x

[156] De Araújo-Filho, H. G., Santos, J. F., Carvalho, M. T. B., Picot, L., Groult, H., Groult, H., Quintans-Júnior, L. J., & Quintans, J. S. (2021). "Anticancer activity of limonene: A systematic review of target signaling pathways." *Phytotherapy Research*, *35*(9), 4957–4970. https://doi.org/10.1002/ptr.7125

[157] Sousa, C., Leitão, A. J., Neves, B. M., Judas, F., Cavaleiro, C., & Mendes, A. M. S. (2020). "Standardised comparison of limonene-derived monoterpenes identifies structural determinants of anti-inflammatory activity." *Scientific Reports*, *10*(1). https://doi.org/10.1038/s41598-020-64032-1

[158] Vieira, A. J., Beserra, F. P., De Souza, M. C., Totti, B., & Rozza, A. L. (2018). "Limonene: Aroma of innovation in health and disease." *Chemico-Biological Interactions*, *283*, 97–106. https://doi.org/10.1016/j.cbi.2018.02.007

[159] D'Alessio, P., Mirshahi, M., Bisson, J., & Béné, M. C. (2014). "Skin repair properties of D-Limonene and perillyl alcohol in murine models." *Anti-inflammatory & Anti-allergy Agents in Medicinal Chemistry*, *13*(1), 29–35. https://doi.org/10.2174/18715230113126660021

[160] Mohammed MSO, Babeanu N, Radu CPCN. "Limonene - A biomolecule with potential applications in regenerative medicinel ". Sci Bull. 2022;XXVI(2): pp. 139–50.

[161] Russo, E. B. (2011). "Taming THC: potential cannabis synergy and phytocannabinoid-terpenoid entourage effects." *British Journal of Pharmacology*, *163*(7), 1344–1364. https://doi.org/10.1111/j.1476-5381.2011.01238.x

[162] Buchbauer, G., Jirovetz, L., Jäger, W., Plank, C., & Dietrich, H. (1993). "Fragrance Compounds and Essential Oils with Sedative Effects upon Inhalation." *Journal of Pharmaceutical Sciences*, *82*(6), 660–664. https://doi.org/10.1002/jps.2600820623

[163] Ghelardini, C., Galeotti, N., Salvatore, G., & Mazzanti, G. (1999). "Local Anaesthetic Activity of the Essential Oil of Lavandula angustifolia." *Planta Medica*, *65*(8), 700–703. https://doi.org/10.1055/s-1999-14045

[164] McPartland, J. M., & Russo, E. B. (2001). "Cannabis and cannabis extracts." *Journal of Cannabis Therapeutics*, *1*(3–4), 103–132. https://doi.org/10.1300/j175v01n03_08

[165] Batista, P., De Paula Werner, M. F., Oliveira, E. C., Burgos, L., Pereira, P., Da Silva Brum, L. F., Story, G. M., & Santos, A. R. (2010). "The antinociceptive effect of (-)-Linalool in models of chronic inflammatory and neuropathic hypersensitivity in mice." *The Journal of Pain*, *11*(11), 1222–1229. https://doi.org/10.1016/j.jpain.2010.02.022

[166] Han, H. D., Cho, Y. J., Cho, S. K., Byeon, Y., Jeon, H. Y., Kim, H. S., Kim, B. G., Bae, D. S., López-Berestein, G., Sood, A. K., Shin, B. C., Park, Y. M., & Lee, J. W. (2016). "Linalool-Incorporated nanoparticles

Phytol

Phytol is commonly found in green tea. It increases GABAergic neurotransmission,[167] exerting a relaxant potential. It also helps in lowering cholesterol.[168]

β-caryophyllene

β-Caryophyllene is found in black pepper, oregano, other edible herbs, green leafy vegetables, and cannabis. It has a hoppy taste and aroma with gastroprotective, anti-inflammatory, analgesic, antifungal, and possibly anticancer properties.[169,170,171] This terpene binds directly to CB2 receptors, which are widely expressed in the immune system. The link with CB2 was documented in 2008 by Swiss scientist Jürg Gertsch, who described β-caryophyllene as a "dietary cannabinoid."[172]

Entourage Effect: Phytopharmaceutical Synergy

In 1998, Israeli scientist Dr. Raphael Mechoulam postulated what is known today as the **entourage effect.** This term describes the effect of all the therapeutic constituents of cannabis acting together,[173] that is, the combination of all the compounds present in the plant is more effective than its isolated elements. The term **full spectrum** is used to describe cannabis-

---

as a novel anticancer agent for epithelial ovarian carcinoma."' *Molecular Cancer Therapeutics, 15*(4), 618–627. https://doi.org/10.1158/1535-7163.mct-15-0733-t

[167] Costa, J. P., Ga, D. O., Aa, D. A., Islam, M. T., Dp, D. S., & Rm, D. F. (2014). "Anxiolytic-like effects of phytol: Possible involvement of GABAergic transmission." *Brain Research, 1547*, 34–42. https://doi.org/10.1016/j.brainres.2013.12.003

[168] Ding, L., Matsumura, M., Obitsu, T., & Sugino, T. (2021). "Phytol supplementation alters plasma concentrations of formate, amino acids, and lipid metabolites in sheep." *Animal, 15*(3), 100174. https://doi.org/10.1016/j.animal.2021.100174

[169] Russo, E. B. (2011). "Taming THC: potential cannabis synergy and phytocannabinoid-terpenoid entourage effects." *British Journal of Pharmacology, 163*(7), 1344–1364. https://doi.org/10.1111/j.1476-5381.2011.01238.x

[170] Eisohly, H. N., Turner, C. E., Clark, A. M., & Eisohly, M. A. (1982). "Synthesis and antimicrobial activities of certain cannabichromene and cannabigerol related compounds." *Journal of Pharmaceutical Sciences, 71*(12), 1319–1323. https://doi.org/10.1002/jps.2600711204

[171] Gertsch, J. (2008). "Antiinflammatory cannabinoids in diet – towards a better understanding of CB2 receptor action?" *Communicative & Integrative Biology, 1*(1), 26–28. https://doi.org/10.4161/cib.1.1.6568

[172] *Ibid.*

[173] Ben-Shabat, S., Fride, E., Sheskin, T., Tamiri, T., Rhee, M. H., Vogel, Z., Bisogno, T., De Petrocellis, L., Di Marzo, V., & Mechoulam, R. (1998). "An entourage effect: inactive endogenous fatty acid glycerol esters enhance 2-arachidonoyl-glycerol cannabinoid activity." *European Journal of Pharmacology, 353*(1), 23–31. https://doi.org/10.1016/s0014-2999(98)00392-6

based medicines that utilize as much or all of the natural therapeutic molecules that the plant has to offer.

The entourage effect is not unique to cannabis, but can be applied to all herbal medicines.

This entourage effect meets the definition of plant protection synergy established by Wagner and Ulrich-Merzenich, who say that for a successful plant protection synergy, four basic theoretical mechanisms must exist:

1. Affect multiple targets within the body;

2. Improve active ingredients absorption;

3. Overcoming bacterial defense mechanisms;

4. Minimize adverse side effects.[174]

The best evidence of the entourage effect comes from renowned cannabis researchers Dr. Mechoulam and Dr. Lester Grinspoon. Dr. Ethan Russo, former US medical consultant at GW Pharmaceuticals, explained the entourage effect in a 2011 article published in *The British Journal of Pharmacology* and reviewed some possible interactions between various cannabinoids and terpenes.[175] The article described a study suggesting that α-pinene may help preserve acetylcholine, which has been implicated in memory formation.[176] Russo suggested that "one of the main side effects of THC is short-term memory impairment... This can be avoided if there is α-pinene in cannabis." Thus, this terpene helps counteract the cognitive impairment that may be associated with THC.[177] Myrcene can reduce resistance in the blood-brain barrier, facilitating the passage of other

---

[174] Wagner, H., & Ulrich-Merzenich, G. (2009). "Synergy research: Approaching a new generation of phytopharmaceuticals." *Phytomedicine, 16*(2–3), 97–110. https://doi.org/10.1016/j.phymed.2008.12.018

[175] Russo, E. B. (2011). "Taming THC: potential cannabis synergy and phytocannabinoid-terpenoid entourage effects." *British Journal of Pharmacology, 163*(7), 1344–1364. https://doi.org/10.1111/j.1476-5381.2011.01238.x

[176] Perry, N. S. L., Houghton, P. J., Theobald, A., Jenner, P., & Perry, E. K. (2000). "In-vitro Inhibition of Human Erythrocyte Acetylcholinesterase by *Salvia lavandulaefolia* Essential Oil and Constituent Terpenes." *Journal of Pharmacy and Pharmacology, 52*(7), 895–902. https://doi.org/10.1211/0022357001774598

[177] Russo, E. B. (2011). "Taming THC: potential cannabis synergy and phytocannabinoid-terpenoid entourage effects." *British Journal of Pharmacology, 163*(7), 1344–1364. https://doi.org/10.1111/j.1476-5381.2011.01238.x

beneficial chemicals.[178] Interestingly, a combination of terpenes, α-pinene, myrcene, and β-caryophyllene helps to reduce anxiety.[179] A mixture of pinene and CBG shows promise in the treatment of methicillin-resistant Staphylococcus aureus,[180] while a combination of linalool, limonene, and CBD has been shown to be an effective acne treatment.[181]

Due to the Schedule I status of the cannabis plant, the US federal government has placed research using natural botanical cannabis out of reach of most scientists. As a result, there is no robust evidence confirming the entourage effect. As with so many aspects of the ECS, cannabis, and cannabinoids, researchers are still only scratching the surface. Some double-blind clinical trials have been conducted to investigate the effects of terpenes, flavonoids, and cannabinoids found in cannabis, but there is still a large knowledge gap waiting to be filled. Future studies are needed to provide more evidence about the entourage effect.

---

[178] Surendran, S., Qassadi, F., Surendran, G., Lilley, D., & Heinrich, M. (2021). "Myrcene—What are the potential health benefits of this flavouring and aroma agent?" *Frontiers in Nutrition, 8.* https://doi.org/10.3389/fnut.2021.699666

[179] Wagner, H., & Ulrich-Merzenich, G. (2009b). "Synergy research: Approaching a new generation of phytopharmaceuticals." *Phytomedicine, 16*(2–3), 97–110. https://doi.org/10.1016/j.phymed.2008.12.018

[180] Appendino, G., Gibbons, S., Giana, A., Pagani, A., Grassi, G., Stavri, M., Smith, E., & Rahman, M. M. (2008). "Antibacterial Cannabinoids from *Cannabis sativa*: A Structure−Activity Study." *Journal of Natural Products, 71*(8), 1427–1430. https://doi.org/10.1021/np8002673

[181] Russo, E. B. (2011). "Taming THC: potential cannabis synergy and phytocannabinoid-terpenoid entourage effects." *British Journal of Pharmacology, 163*(7), 1344–1364. https://doi.org/10.1111/j.1476-5381.2011.01238.x

Part II: Cannabis Use & Side Effects

This section provides insight and guidance on information that is typically available for other medications such as dosage, routes of administration, side effects, dependence, metabolism, toxicology, pregnancy, and considerations for driving.

Dosing

Since the 1980s, breeders and cultivators have diligently worked to maximize THC production in the cannabis plant. The THC content of cannabis flowers in commercial dispensaries can be up to about 30% or more and 90% or higher in full-spectrum extractions.

The concentration of each of the over 512 molecular constituents in cannabis varies from one variety to another and even from plant to plant within the same family. Unlike pharmaceutical medicines, the cannabis plant is a living organism with unique DNA from seed to seed. The end product concentrations result from nature (the plant's genetics) and nurture (the plant's growing conditions). Additionally, chemical content varies not only by variety but also from flower to flower on a living plant, accounting for such details as the distance from its light source and the type of lighting used.

Like other herbal medicaments, dosage is often most effectively measured through titration. Titration means starting with small doses and waiting to feel the effects before deciding if a larger dose can be tolerated. Patients feel the effects of inhaled cannabis more immediately, although the dosage is much more challenging to measure. For other routes of ingestion, titration should start at 1–2 milligrams of THC and the patient should wait at least 90 minutes before attempting to increase the dose.

Investigational New Drug (IND) Program

The federal cannabis treatment program is a practical, contemporary basis for speculation regarding dosage. The Investigational New Drug (IND) program started in 1978 with a single glaucoma patient, Robert Randall, as a result of a legal agreement to preserve Randall's eyesight by allowing him to legally use cannabis to lower his intraocular pressure. At first, the cannabis was sent to Johns Hopkins, and an assistant professor monitored Randall's use. When the professor moved on to another institution, the government was finally forced, by a historic 1978 court decision, to provide Randall with his sight-saving cannabis. This judicial decree established the Investigational New Drug program.

The IND provided Randall, and subsequently 14 other patients, the amount of cannabis necessary to obtain a therapeutic result for their medical conditions.

The program was closed to new participants and terminated in 1992, but the 15 patients who were already part of the program were grandfathered in for life. The federal government provides seven to nine pounds of cannabis cigarettes per year to IND patients. As of early 2024, the federal government still supplies four patients every month with 300 4% THC cannabis cigarettes, each containing nine-tenths of a gram of ground cannabis flowers.[182]

In 2004, Dr. Ethan Russo and Mary Lynn Mathre, RN, did a comprehensive health study of the history and physical status of four of the then-seven surviving IND patients. Other than their underlying medical problem for which they were taking cannabis to treat, they were in normal health for people of their ages and genders.[183]

Here is information on three of the IND patients:

Age/Gender	Qualifying Condition	IND Approval- Years of Cannabis Usage	Daily Cannabis/THC Content
62, female	Glaucoma	(1988) 39 years	8 grams (0.28 oz), 3.8%
52, male	Nail-Patella Syndrome	(1989) 41 years	7 grams (0.25 oz), 3.75%
48, female	Multiple Sclerosis	(1989) 41 years	9 grams (0.32 oz), 3.5%

How to Dose Raw Cannabis Flowers and Botanicals

THC dosage in raw cannabis flowers can be reasonably determined with simple math; one gram (1000 mg) of cannabis containing 10% THC has 100 mg of THC. This, however, is not the amount that is delivered to the patient when cannabis is smoked because **pyrolysis** destroys 70% of available THC. Therefore, when smoked, a cannabis cigarette delivers no more than 30% of

---

[182] Russo, Ethan, Mary Lynn Mathre, Al Byrne, Robert Velin, et al. "Chronic Cannabis Use in the Compassionate Investigational New Drug Program: An Examination of Benefits and Adverse Effects of Legal Clinical Cannabis." *Journal of Cannabis Therapeutics* 2(1), 2002

[183] Roffman, R.A. and R. Stephens, eds. "Cannabis Dependence: Its Nature, Consequences, and Treatment." Cambridge University Press, 2006.

the THC it contains to the bloodstream. An additional amount is lost to the air, and still more is left in the ash, so only about 16-17% is absorbed.[184] Inhaled cannabis is more efficient than orally consumed cannabis for immediate relief of nausea or pain, despite the wasted THC from smoking.[185] It takes 45 to 75 minutes for THC to reach therapeutic levels in the bloodstream when ingested orally, and 85% of THC is metabolized through the liver on the first pass to the very psychotropic 11-hydroxy-THC.

Isolated THC and CBD Medicines

Some patients have found that either THC or CBD alone can be effective therapeutic agents; however, they are rarely, if ever, as effective as the two together. There are several prescription THC-only medicines on the market, including Marinol (dronabinol) and Cesamet (nabilone). These are legal, FDA-approved pharmaceuticals that contain only synthetic THC. They are approved to ease cancer treatment-related nausea and appetite suppression. Not surprisingly, these synthetic THC pharmaceuticals are more expensive than cannabis, do not work as well, and have more side effects. They do not benefit from the entourage effect but do have therapeutic applications.

Clinical experts recommend using a full spectrum extract rather than a single isolate such as CBD or THC because of growing evidence supporting the entourage effect.[186] Even very low amounts of THC can contribute to beneficial medical effects. In most instances, the therapeutic benefits of CBD are enhanced by using 1-2 mg of THC. This THC dose does not produce euphoria.

Physicians and patients need to guard against "**euphoriphobia**." Many are adamant about not wanting to feel "high." While the reason for having such a feeling may be from a bad experience in the past, such as paranoia or anxiety, this usually stems from an instance of ingesting too much THC.

Dose Experience with Patent Medicines

Some light may be shed on appropriate contemporary dosing by looking at the doses recommended in cannabis-containing **patent medicines** popular

---

[184] House of Lords. "Science of Technology - Ninth Report." United Kingdom Parliament. November 4, 1998.

[185] Pharmacopeia, United States. "11th rev." http://antiquecannabisbook.com/Appendix/USP1942.htm/.

[186] Russo, E. B. (2019). "The case for the entourage effect and conventional breeding of clinical cannabis: No 'Strain,' no gain." *Frontiers in Plant Science, 9*. https://doi.org/10.3389/fpls.2018.01969

in the late 19th century and early 20th century. In the early years of the 20th century, cannabis was widely available as a medical treatment. It was used as a nerve sedative and an analgesic, prescribed for migraine, neuralgia, and dysmenorrhea, among other indications. The preparations available were an alcoholic tincture and aqueous extract.

The suggested doses were:

- **Novice user**: 2.5–5 mg
- **Experienced or moderate user**: 10–20 mg
- **Heavy or frequent user**: 25 mg+

As little as 2.5 to 5 mg THC can cause euphoria or dysphoria for a small percentage of the population. For most users, about 10 mg of THC can cause feelings of euphoria. **Tolerance** to euphoria can develop, so it may not occur for heavy users, even with much higher dosages. For novice users, starting with the respiratory route of administration is best due to the relative ease of dose titration. Start with a low dose and slowly increase it to find the dose that balances the desired therapeutic effect against any undesirable side effects.

Therapeutic Dose

It is difficult to stand on firm ground when determining the appropriate cannabis dosage for a specific condition due to the lack of double-blind studies and confounded by plant and human variability. The basis for speculation on dosage estimates and cannabinoid ratios is derived from current research, animal and tissue culture studies, plus clinical experience. Many questions still need to be more thoroughly answered through clinical studies.

When it comes to dosing, physicians are left with relying on research done with products such as Marinol, Epidiolex, and Sativex and must base their findings on the experience of patients and healthcare professionals. Such practitioners include MDs, DOs, naturopaths, nurse practitioners, and nutritionists. Private and publicly funded research is still in its infancy. The federal government is still primarily focused on studying single molecules and is not particularly supportive of the studies necessary to fully understand plant-based medicine.

There are several cannabinoid and cannabis-based prescription medicines on the global market today. These include dronabinol and Nabilone. Nabiximols (Sativex) is approved for medical use in 24 countries and is a full-spectrum alcohol extract. Experience with these standardized cannabis and cannabinoid prescription preparations provides some guidance for the dosage of cannabis.

Respiratory Dose

There is no "one size fits all" dose. An effective dose of THC is usually considered to be between 2 to 40 mg when smoked and between 20 to 90 mg when taken orally.[187] Clinical experience has demonstrated that with a 20 mg dose of dronabinol, at least 30% of patients complain of **dysphoria**. For many conditions, a dose of cannabis that contains 2-5 mg THC is a good starting point and is usually sufficient to obtain the desired therapeutic effect without the dose generating euphoria.

Under normal smoking conditions, 16-19% of the THC in the cannabis cigarette is consumed. The rest is pyrolyzed (burned) and wafts off in smoke. Smoking burns (oxidizes) the molecules in cannabis, which creates additional molecules to inhale besides just those produced naturally by the plant, and some of these are chemical constituents that can irritate the bronchial tree and/or are carcinogenic.

The respiratory route can also be achieved by vaporization. Vaporization (heating volatile oils until they enter the gas phase) delivers 70% fewer irritants to the bronchial tree and lungs than pyrolysis. Vaporized cannabis does not produce the oxidized compounds and carcinogens created by the combustion effect from smoking.

Oral Dose

Clinical experience prescribing THC (dronabinol) provides a guide to dose ranges for many conditions. Dronabinol can be used as a guide for the doctor and patient for a more specific starting dose range of THC when beginning use with botanical cannabis. Information from using nabiximols (Sativex), a widely studied, full-spectrum alcohol extract with a 1:1 THC to CBD ratio, also provides evidence clinicians can utilize.

---

[187] Noyes, Russell, S. Brunk, David A. Baram, and Arthur Canter. "Analgesic Effect of Delta-9-Tetrahydrocannabinol." *The Journal of Clinical Pharmacology* 15, no. 2-3 (1975): 139-

Analgesic Dose

Research by Noyes et al. in the 1970s found that 20 mg of THC was the therapeutic equivalent of 60 mg of codeine, which suggests it would benefit patients experiencing physical pain.[188] Clinicians utilizing cannabinoid medicine find that cannabis containing 10-20 mg THC per dose, plus an equal or lesser amount of CBD, is often helpful for relieving pain, as many terpenes have anti-inflammatory properties. For **analgesia**, start with a cannabis product containing 10 mg of THC and 10 mg CBD, taken three to four times daily. Then, if there are no adverse side effects but little to no pain relief response, raise the dosage to 15 mg THC and 15 mg CBD. Deborah Malka, MD, PhD, recommends never using more than a 1:1 ratio of THC to CBD for pain relief. Sativex, a 1:1 THC to CBD tincture, has been shown in clinical trials to treat intractable pain.

Anxiety Relief Dose

Administering relatively low doses of THC (in the 2.5-5 mg range two to three times daily), usually combined with CBD, can work to control not only anxiety but also some of the symptoms of autism spectrum disorder, social anxiety, ADD, ADHD, and PTSD. A patient can utilize two to four times the amount of CBD as THC for anxiety relief, so 5-10 mg CBD is fine, as many terpenes also have anti-anxiety properties.

Treating Cancer

There are several constituents of cannabis, including CBN, CBC, CBG, THC, THCa, and CBD, that have been identified as having cancer cell-killing properties. A combination of the plant's constituents is often superior to isolated compounds. Cannabinoids possess synergistic anti-cancer properties. Cannabis can induce **apoptosis** in cancer cells, prevent the proliferation of cancer cells, suppress tumor angiogenesis, and inhibit cancer adhesion and migration.

The dosages suggested to kill cancer cells are quite high. Most patients will experience dysphoria for at least ten days and, in many cases, even longer. According to Dustin Sulak, DO, the goal is 5-25 mg per kg per day, total cannabinoids divided TID-QID.

Due to legal constraints and a lack of clinical trials, such cancer treatment is

---

[188] Ibid.

usually provided only by lay healers. While each lay healer has their own slightly different, unique approach, the range is two to three grams per day of concentrated cannabis for 60-90 days, followed by a lifetime maintenance dose of 0.5 to 1 gram per day of concentrated cannabis.

Evidence of cancer treatment can be found in **full extract cannabis oil** (FECO, aka Rick Simpson Oil or **RSO**). **FECO** is used by lay healers who often start with a kilogram (2.2 pounds) of cannabis and perform an alcohol extraction before purging off the solvent, resulting in thick, concentrated oil. Each lay healer has their own protocol for making and dosing the oil, leading to a variety of dosages. The recommended usage is usually some variant of one to three grams per day of FECO for 60 or 90 days. Joe Goldstrich, MD, provides an excellent overview of lay practices and current research regarding dosage and phytochemical content in *The Cannabis-Cancer Connection* (Flower Valley Press, 2023).

Not surprisingly, it is common for cancer patients treated with high-THC cannabis to report an unpleasant effect beyond euphoria to dysphoria and describe the effects specifically as anxiety and/or paranoia. While the side effects from cannabis are not as significant as those from conventional chemotherapy and radiation, cannabis, especially in high doses, has some genuine side effects, including nausea, vomiting, anxiety, dysphoria, panic attacks, and paranoia. There are several strategies for mitigating the side effects of the cannabis dose needed to treat cancer. *See Side Effects of Cannabis.*

Other Dosage Studies

The following are some examples of various studies done using dronabinol that show the variability of a "standard" dose. These studies are consistent in that a standard dose of dronabinol (synthetic THC) ranges from 2.5 up to 15 mg per square meter of body surface, taken four to six times a day.

Spasticity

Cannabis has been shown to aid in the reduction of spasticity (tightness and stiffness in muscles) in people with multiple sclerosis (MS). The late Dr. J. Thomas Ungerleider of UCLA led a study on the effects of cannabis on spasticity using doses of 2.5-15 mg of THC. He found that a dose of over 7.5 mg showed significant improvement. Ungerleider et al. demonstrated an apparent dose-related reduction of spasticity with 7.5–15 mg THC.[189] Another study found that 10 mg of THC reduced spasticity.[190] Also, GW Pharmaceuticals (now Jazz Pharmaceuticals) in England has had excellent results in treating spasticity and pain related to MS with nabiximols. The doses being used in these trials are, or at least were, proprietary information according to GW Pharmaceuticals's US legal counsel, Alice Mead, formerly of the California Medical Association (CMA).[191]

Seizures

In a double-blind clinical trial of CBD, Cunha et al. found cannabis to be effective in abolishing or reducing seizures in seven out of eight subjects, each receiving 100 mg daily, whereas only one out of seven placebo controls reported any improvement. The conclusion was that CBD had a beneficial effect on patients who have secondary generalized epilepsy and did not benefit from known antiepileptic drugs.[192]

---

[189] Ungerleider, J. Thomas, Therese Andyrsiak, Lynn Fairbanks, George W. Ellison, and Lawrence W. Myers. "Delta-9-THC in the treatment of spasticity associated with multiple sclerosis." *Advances in Alcohol & Substance Abuse* 7, no. 1 (1988): 39-50.

[190] Petro, Denis J., and C. Ellenberger. "Treatment of Human Spasticity with Δ^9-Tetrahydrocannabinol." *The Journal of Clinical Pharmacology* 21, no. S1 (1981).

[191] Novotna, A., J. Mares, S. Ratcliffe, I. Novakova, M. Vachova, O. Zapletalova, C. Gasperini et al. "A randomized, double-blind, placebo-controlled, parallel-group, enriched-design study of nabiximols (Sativex®), as add-on therapy, in subjects with refractory spasticity caused by multiple sclerosis." *European Journal of Neurology* 18, no. 9 (2011): 1122-1131.

[192] Cunha, Jomar M., E. A. Carlini, Aparecido E. Pereira, Oswaldo L. Ramos, Camilo Pimentel, Rubens Gagliardi, W. L. Sanvito, N. Lander, and R. Mechoulam. "Chronic administration of cannabidiol to healthy volunteers and epileptic patients." *Pharmacology* 21, no. 3 (1980): 175-185.

The following chart provides rough dosage guidelines by condition based on available studies:

Anxiety	Full spectrum extract containing 2.5-5 mg 1:1 THC to CBD
Nausea	2.5-5 mg dronabinol or a similar dose of THC contained in a full spectrum extract.
Insomnia	5-10 mg of THC from an entire plant vaporized or smoked to go to sleep, 5-10 mg of THC (dronabinol) or edible at bedtime to maintain sleep, may add 5-15 mg of CBD.
Pain	15-30 mg or more of THC with a similar amount of CBD. CBD decreases possible dysphoria and is also helpful in cases of inflammation.
Autism Spectrum Disorder	This varies enormously, from 2.5-5 mg of THC to two-three times a day to as much as 35 mg of CBD alone. There is wide variability in the THC-to-CBD ratio.
Seizures	While full spectrum high CBD extract is popular, as is CBD alone, there is compelling research and historical evidence that THC plays a vital role in controlling epilepsy. Relatively low doses of cannabis, as infrequently as once a day, have proven effective in decreasing seizure frequency; however, a somewhat higher dose may be necessary.
Cancer	Dr. Donald Abrams, an oncologist at UCSF School of Medicine, has said there is enough basic scientific evidence and anecdotal reports to justify a double-blind study. One such study was conducted in the United Kingdom using 25 mg THC and 25 mg CBD on glioblastoma patients. The treated groups had a 40% increase in survival time.[193] Lay healers often use 2-6x that dose.

---

[193] Donald Abrams, M.D., "Marijuana for Medical Professionals Presentation," Denver, 2017.

Routes of Administration

Different effects can result from the varied routes of administration when consuming cannabis. Each option gives patients more control over administration and the following results. The two main routes are through inhalation and ingestion. When inhaled, THC enters capillaries in the lungs and alveoli, passes into general circulation through the pulmonary veins, and quickly crosses the blood-brain barrier. This method sends THC to the brain without going through the liver. However, when ingested orally, THC is absorbed in the small intestine and is then carried to the liver in the blood, where it is metabolized by subclasses of cytochrome P450 (abbreviated CYP), specifically the CYP2C and CYP3A enzymes. About 85% of the THC is metabolized to 11-hydroxy-THC, which is more psychotropic (inebriating) than THC.

The following is a list of routes of administration and the considerations for choosing each:

- **Smoking**: The most efficient and quickest-acting route, but it can irritate the bronchial tree.
- **Vaporizing**: This route produces 70% fewer irritants and preserves more cannabinoids and terpenes than **combustion** (smoking).
- **Water Pipe (Bong)**: Removes irritants and THC equally and cools smoke.
- **Sublingual**: **Tinctures** applied under the tongue act in about 15 minutes.
- **Tea**: A traditional form of ingestion (used for millennia in India). It can be made from leaves, roots, or flowering tops of the plant. Tea is usually made with milk or cream to bind to fat-soluble cannabinoids.
- **Oral/Edibles**: On average, these take 45 to 75 minutes to act. Read the label to avoid taking too high a dose.
- **Topical**: Used for over a century by curanderos in Southern Mexico and Central America to treat arthritis in hands and wrists.
- **Prescription**: Marinol (dronabinol, THC), nabiximols (Sativex) (approved in Canada, UK, NZ, and EU), Cannabidiol (Epidiolex), approved for sale in the US.
- **Rectal**: Full Extract Cannabis Oil (FECO) **suppositories** can be used to decrease dysphoria.

- **Juicing**: Raw, freshly picked, undried flowers and leaves contain all of the plant's cannabinoids in the acid form, including THCa (the non-psychotropic precursor to THC), CBDa, etc. There are limited or no psychotropic effects from juicing a freshly picked cannabis plant.

Oral Ingestion

This is one of the oldest known routes of administration, having been used in India as bhang tea since at least 1100 BCE. The drink must contain a form of fat, such as dairy, to capture the fat-soluble (lipophilic) molecules in cannabis. Oral tinctures are widely used, such as in prescription nabiximols and in flavored drinks to which cannabis has been added. Oral ingestion results in a longer length of action and is helpful in treating chronic, omnipresent conditions like Crohn's Disease or rheumatoid arthritis. Still, it can be disconcerting if the ingested dose is too high and leads to dysphoria.

As dosing becomes more precise, this problem of consuming an unknown dose of THC is becoming less common. More edibles have dosages on their labels, and cannabis consumers are better able to measure an appropriate amount for themselves. Furthermore, there has been an increase in the therapeutic use of high CBD and low THC products, allowing for more variety in dosages.

A Standardized Cannabis Medicine: Nabiximols

GW Pharmaceuticals, now owned by Jazz Pharmaceuticals, has dealt with the issue of standardization and reproducible therapeutic results by creating Sativex™ (nabiximols), a full spectrum, alcohol-extracted cannabis tincture. Sativex™ is produced through a proprietary recipe using standardized monocropped (cloned) plants. The company initially had six greenhouses in an old munitions factory in southern England. Each greenhouse in use by GW is home to a different variety of cannabis and contains 10,000 plants. This growing process ensures the consistency of plant material suitable for standardized pharmaceutical products.

The prescription pharmaceutical product nabiximols is made from the flowering tops of multiple plants, thus further standardizing the product. It is composed of a 50/50 combination of two cultivars of cannabis: one high in THC and the other high in CBD. Nabiximols is a liquid that is administered sublingually by a metered dose inhaler. In 2014, GW introduced Epidiolex™, a high CBD, low THC, full spectrum extract for the treatment of epileptic seizures.[194] Extensive studies have been done by GW Pharmaceuticals showing that their tincture of cannabis is much less psychotropic than dronabinol, which is a THC-only product.[195] Nabiximols is legal to prescribe in 24 countries. However, despite successful phase III clinical trials for treating intractable pain in upstate New York in 2011, the United States is not yet one of them. Epidiolex (cannabidiol) was approved in June 2018.

Marinol™ (Dronabinol) / Syndros™

In 1985, the federal government approved the sale of dronabinol, synthetic Δ^9-THC capsules—trade name Marinol™. Marinol comes in 2.5, 5, and 10 mg doses. After oral administration, dronabinol has an onset of action of approximately 30 minutes to one hour and a peak effect at 2-4 hours. Duration of action for psychotropic effects, if they are present, is 4 to 6 hours, but the appetite stimulant effect of dronabinol may continue for 24 hours or longer after administration. A recently approved variation is Syndros™, dronabinol in variable doses delivered orally via a needleless syringe.

Why is nabiximols less of a euphoriant than dronabinol? There are at least two reasons: First, nabiximols is liquid cannabis (a mixture of two full spectrum alcohol extracts), and therefore, the entourage effect is present. The presence of hundreds of cannabinoids, particularly CBD, and over 200 terpenes makes it more effective than dronabinol and has fewer side effects. Second, dronabinol contains only THC, the principal euphoriant in cannabis, and does not contain CBD, meaning dronabinol is more likely to cause dysphoria than cannabis. There are no other cannabinoids present in dronabinol, eliminating the possibility of engaging the entourage effect. There is no CBD present to help block out the intoxicating effect of THC.

Most patients tolerate 2.5 to 5 mg doses of dronabinol with little or no euphoria. At 10 mg, a small percentage of patients will begin to feel dysphoric side effects. The percentage of patients with complaints of dysphoria increases at 15 mg. This side effect is less likely to occur with full-spectrum cannabis that contains CBD. While CBD partially blocks THC euphoria, the euphoria can still occur. Always start low with the dose of THC and increase

---

[194] "History and Approach." GW Pharmaceuticals. Last modified 2016 https://www.gwpharm.com/about-us/history-approach/.

[195] Robson, Philip. "Abuse potential and psychoactive effects of d-9-tetrahydrocannabinol and cannabidiol oromucosal spray (Sativex), a new cannabinoid medicine." Expert Opinion on Drug Safety 10, no. 5 (2011): 675-685.

slowly.

Side Effects of Marinol® (Dronabinol)

The Physician's Desk Reference (PDR) contains the side effects and warnings for most of today's manufactured prescription drugs within its hundreds of pages. These synthetically manufactured medications often have more significant side effects than plant-based medicines. There are several adverse side effects experienced by patients who consume dronabinol.

Dronabinol contains only THC and is manufactured without the other 512 molecules found within cannabis, which would balance and control its psychotropic effects. Dronabinol is more expensive, has more side effects, and doesn't work as well as cannabis. Some of dronabinol's adverse effects include dizziness, drowsiness, hyperemesis, nausea, and seizures. On the other hand, it has considerable off-label effective uses, and several alternative reasons exist to prescribe it.

The FDA's rescheduling of synthetic THC, Marinol (dronabinol), attests to the safety of cannabis. The FDA rarely moves a drug to a lower schedule. In the case of THC, the most psychotropic constituent of cannabis, Marinol was moved from Schedule II to Schedule III, where it remains to this day. The entire cannabis plant, if it contains less than 0.3% THC, is now considered legal hemp, yet botanical cannabis remains a Schedule I drug with no accepted medical use. Interestingly, botanical cannabis has fewer side effects than Marinol.

Juicing

Juicing the raw leaves and consuming the juice doesn't produce euphoria because all the cannabinoids in the raw plant are in the acid form (have a carboxyl group). There are trace levels of THC in raw cannabis, but non-psychotropic THCa is the dominant cannabinoid. For THCa to lead to euphoria, it needs to be decarboxylated into THC through heating. Juicing allows the use of high doses of non-psychotropic cannabinoid acids. When eaten, vaporized, or smoked, higher doses of decarboxylated cannabis can often cause unpleasant euphoria, dysphoria, **hyperemesis**, and/or panic attacks. Higher doses are required for the use of cannabis as an anti-proliferative agent.

William Courtney, MD, is the world's leading juicing proponent. He recommends that his patients mix the cannabis juice (1 part) with carrot juice (10 parts) to counteract the bitterness and drink the mixture three times a day. Dr. Courtney suggests that the cannabis plant has the highest CBD content between 70-90 days after sowing. After 90 days, they rapidly produce more THC.[196] Potential conditions that may benefit from raw cannabis include autoimmune disorders, inflammatory disorders, and possibly various types of cancer or precancerous dysplasia.

Inhalation

Smoking cannabis is associated with increased cough, sputum production, and bronchial irritation, but conspicuously not cancer. The benefits of the respiratory route are the rapid onset and the ability to titrate the dosage. Migraines, social anxiety, nausea, seizures, and asthma are conditions where rapid onset is beneficial.

---

[196] "The Importance of THC free Cannabis." *Cannabis Digest*. https://cannabisdigest.ca/importance-thc-free-cannabis/.

Inhalation Methods

Vaporizing	This method heats cannabis to a vaporization point but below the point of combustion. **Vaporization** does not burn the plant material but releases the volatile oils into the air. This results in roughly 70% less irritation to the bronchial tree than traditional smoking. This process still provides rapid onset and the ability to titrate dosage. There are individual vaporizers, like e-cigarettes, and less portable table vaporizers, like the Volcano.
Water Pipe (Bong)	This device uses water to cool and filter the smoke. It not only filters out bronchial irritants but also THC and other plant constituents in the same proportions. The water traps a percentage of the toxins, carcinogens, and pyrolysis byproducts.
Dabbing	**Dabbing** is a form of vaporization that uses a torch to heat a glass, ceramic, or titanium element to vaporize a small amount (or "dab") of cannabis concentrate for inhalation. Oregon Health and Sciences University studied the temperatures used during dabbing and found that the concentrates could become carcinogenic when the heating element was heated over 750°F (399°C). The material released benzene, a known carcinogen, when heated over 950°F (510°C). More equipment and tools have been released onto this market to keep temperatures below 600°F (315.5°C), which is not known to release carcinogens and preserves more of the available terpenes. This is referred to as "low-temp" dabbing.

Understanding Vaping Associated Pulmonary Injury (VAPI)

In 2019, thousands of hospitalizations resulted almost entirely from vape products purchased on the illegal or bootleg markets. By early 2020, 64 people had died of Vaping Associated Pulmonary Injury (VAPI). While many of the deaths have now been linked to a "cutting agent," vitamin E acetate, others have pointed to flavors used in tobacco and cannabis vaping pens. This epidemic continues to expose the numerous flaws in research and regulation of vaporizing products. Vaporizing with equipment that allows for controlled temperature settings with the use of raw cannabis flowers and clean extracts enables users to access the medical efficacy of the vaping route without exposing themselves to the dangers of these unregulated products.

Pesticides

Some states do not strictly regulate pesticides used to cultivate cannabis. While some cannabis is grown in clean, organic, and natural settings, patients using cannabis grown with pesticides are ingesting more than just cannabinoids, terpenes, and other natural plant compounds. Pesticides are neurotoxic.

A study of cannabis extracts by *The Oregonian* newspaper found that some pesticides survived butane and carbon dioxide extraction processes and were concentrated into the product.[197] Although the concentration was too low to detect on the raw flowers, the byproduct, when concentrated, was not. Not all labs are testing correctly to prevent this problem, so there may be products on legal shelves that say they are pesticide-free but are not.

Topical

Topical application of cannabis tinctures has been used for arthritis pain relief for over 100 years by Curanderos, lay healers, in Southern Mexico and Central America. The topical application of cannabis salves is helpful for the relief of arthritic pain close to the body's surface, such as in the fingers or wrists. Topical application can also promote the relief of muscle spasms, particularly in the trapezius. It also can help treat numerous skin conditions. Topical CBD is an anti-inflammatory, and THC is an analgesic. Several terpenes also have anti-inflammatory and/or analgesic effects. Using topical applications does not result in a psychotropic effect.

Metabolism

Cannabis and cannabinoids are metabolized by the cytochrome P450 (CYP) enzyme system. The CYP system contributes to the metabolism of drugs by

---

[197] Crombie, N. (n.d.). *Marijuana and pesticides*. OregonLive.com.
https://www.oregonlive.com/projects/marijuana-legalization/pesticides/index.html

oxidizing them, which generally means incorporating an oxygen atom into the drug's molecular structure. Oxidation usually makes a compound more water-soluble and, therefore, easier for the kidneys to filter out.

CBD and other plant cannabinoids have the potential to inhibit or increase the plasma levels of many pharmaceuticals by inhibiting or activating the activity of the CYP enzymes.[198] This enzyme group metabolizes most drugs. In insufficient dosages, CBD can temporarily deactivate CYP enzymes,[199] which alters the metabolism of many compounds, including THC.

Certain compounds in grapefruit can inhibit the expression of some CYP enzymes. CBD is a more potent inhibitor of CYP enzymes than the grapefruit compound bergapten, the strongest of several grapefruit components that inhibit CYPs, also known to give bergamot tea its distinctive smell and flavor.[200]

CBD reduces the enzymatic degradation of Warfarin, thereby increasing its duration of action and effect. A person taking a CBD-rich product should seek the advice of their physician. If the patient takes blood thinners, checking clotting time and adjusting dosage accordingly is necessary.

THC is soluble in lipids and can be quickly absorbed by adipose (fatty) tissue when it enters the bloodstream. On its first pass through the liver, 85% of THC is metabolized to 11-hydroxy-THC (11-OH-THC).[201] This metabolite significantly contributes to psychotropic effects. It can activate the CB1 receptor in the brain and produce euphoria with greater potency than its precursor. After being absorbed by fatty tissue, THC gradually returns to the bloodstream, going to the liver to be metabolized and eliminated in urine and feces.[202] With frequent use, THC tends to accumulate in fatty tissue and the

---

[198] Watanabe, Kazuhito, Satoshi Yamaori, Tatsuya Funahashi, Toshiyuki Kimura, and Ikuo Yamamoto. "Cytochrome P450 enzymes involved in the metabolism of tetrahydrocannabinols and cannabinol by human hepatic microsomes." *Life Sciences* 80, no. 15 (2007): 1415-1419

[199] Stout, Stephen M., and Nina M. Cimino. "Exogenous cannabinoids as substrates, inhibitors, and inducers of human drug metabolizing enzymes: a systematic review." *Drug Metabolism Reviews* 46, no. 1 (2014): 86-95.

[200] Jiang, Rongrong, Satoshi Yamaori, Shuso Takeda, Ikuo Yamamoto, and Kazuhito Watanabe. "Identification of 61cytochrome P450 enzymes responsible for metabolism of cannabidiol by human liver microsomes." *Life Sciences* 89, no. 5-6 (2011): 165-170.

[201] Lemberger, L. (1973, January 1). "Tetrahydrocannabinol Metabolism In Man". *Drug Metabolism & Disposition*. https://dmd.aspetjournals.org/content/1/1/461/tab-article-info

[202] Chayasirisobhon, S. (2021). "Mechanisms of action and pharmacokinetics of cannabis." *The Permanente Journal*, 25(1), 1–3. https://doi.org/10.7812/tpp/19.200

liver. After a week, THC is still present in the blood but drops below the level of detection, and the non-psychotropic metabolite, 9-carboxy-THC, is present in concentrated form in the urine for weeks. Thus, in regular cannabis users, THC metabolites can still be found in the urine weeks after the last use.

Half-Life/Length of Effect

Because THC is fat soluble when it enters the bloodstream, it is rapidly absorbed by **adipose tissue** (half-life: 30 minutes). On its first pass through the liver, 85% of THC is metabolized to 11-hydroxy-THC (11-OH-THC). This metabolite contributes significantly to the psychotropic effects of cannabis. It activates the CB1 cannabinoid receptor in the brain and produces euphoria, which is greater than the parent compound, Δ^9- THC.

After being promptly absorbed into the body fat, the THC then gradually returns osmotically to the bloodstream, where it goes to the liver, is metabolized, and is eliminated in urine and feces (half-life: a few days.). With repeated use, THC tends to accumulate in adipose tissue and the liver. THC itself has been found in blood toxicology screens up to a week after the last use in a regular consumer. After a week, THC is still in the blood but falls below the detection level, and a non-psychotropic metabolite 9-carboxy-THC is still present to be concentrated in the urine. As a result, in regular consumers of cannabis, THC metabolites can still be found in the urine weeks after the last use.

Onset of Effects

When smoked, the acute effects of cannabis begin within a few minutes. The plasma concentration peaks after seven to 10 minutes, but the peak effect is usually felt after 20–30 minutes. Some effects may last for two to three hours. When consumed orally, cannabis takes effect 45 minutes to two hours after consumption, and the therapeutic effects, as well as "the high," can last from three to eight hours.

Drug Interactions

To date, the clinical impact of many of the potential drug interactions with cannabinoids is unknown. Theoretically, any drug that interacts with the CYP enzymes (isoforms 3A4, 2C19, 2C9, 2C8/9), UGT (1A9, 2B7), BCRP, BSEP, and

CES1 presents a risk of interaction with cannabinoids.[203,204] In general, drugs metabolized by these enzymes increase substrate-associated side effects, inhibitors would increase cannabinoid effects and bioavailability, and inducers would decrease it.[205,206] These enzymes are part of the metabolism of many drugs, increasing the potential for drug interaction, which, if not considered in the management of the dose and follow-up, can have unexpected consequences for the patient's health.

Despite possible interactions, some combinations do not appear to have clinically relevant consequences. For example, in the case of patients with HIV undergoing treatment with various antiretroviral drugs (drugs with potential interaction with cannabinoids), no worsening of the immune status was observed when treated with cannabis for therapeutic purposes. However, viral load and immune status are advisable.[207] Another example where theory does not match practice is in the case of chemotherapy, as cannabinoids have not shown clinically relevant interactions.[208]

Medication that has the potential to raise liver aminotransferases, such as statins, cannabis, and cannabinoids, may increase the risk of liver complications. Cannabinoids have been associated on numerous occasions with hepatotoxicity; therefore, it is advisable to monitor liver function when there is a risk of this kind of drug interaction.[209,210] Furthermore, one can

---

[203] Qian, Y., Gurley, B. J., & Markowitz, J. S. (2019). "The potential for pharmacokinetic interactions between cannabis products and conventional medications." *Journal of Clinical Psychopharmacology*, 39(5), 462–471. https://doi.org/10.1097/jcp.0000000000001089

[204] Buchtová, T., Lukac, D. M., Škrott, Z., Chroma, K., Bártek, J., & Mistrík, M. (2023). "Drug–Drug Interactions of Cannabidiol with Standard-of-Care Chemotherapeutics." *International Journal of Molecular Sciences*, 24(3), 2885. https://doi.org/10.3390/ijms24032885

[205] Stout, S. M., & Cimino, N. M. (2013). "Exogenous cannabinoids as substrates, inhibitors, and inducers of human drug metabolizing enzymes: a systematic review." *Drug Metabolism Reviews*, 46(1), 86–95. https://doi.org/10.3109/03602532.2013.849268

[206] Qian, Y., Gurley, B. J., & Markowitz, J. S. (2019b). "The potential for pharmacokinetic interactions between cannabis products and conventional medications." *Journal of Clinical Psychopharmacology*, 39(5), 462–471. https://doi.org/10.1097/jcp.0000000000001089

[207] Abrams DI, Hilton JF, Leiser RJ, Shade SB, Elbeik TA, Aweeka FT, et al. "Short-term effects of cannabinoids in patients with HIV-1 infection: a randomized, placebo-controlled clinical trial." *Ann Intern Med*. 2003 Aug;139(4):258–66.

[208] Bouquie R, Guillaume D, Mazare H, Cogne M, Mahé J, Grégoire M, et al. "Cannabis and anticancer drugs: societal usage and expected pharmacological interactions – a review." *Fundam Clin Pharmacol*. 2018;32(5):462–84.

[209] Borini P, Guimarães RC, Borini SB. "Possible hepatotoxicity of chronic marijuana usage." *Sao Paulo Med J Rev* Paul Med. 2004 May;122(3):110–6.

[210] Thiele EA, Marsh ED, French JA, Mazurkiewicz MB, Benbadis SR, Joshi C, et al. "Cannabidiol in patients with seizures associated with Lennox-Gastaut syndrome (GWPCARE4): a randomised, double-blind, placebo-controlled phase 3 trial." *Lancet*. 2018;391(10125):1085–96.

consider reducing the cannabinoid dose to half the conventional dose, increasing it slowly and gradually up to half the maximum dose.[211]

Other medications that require caution are sedatives. Patients treated with benzodiazepines and opioids may experience an additive effect on sedation when treated with cannabinoids. In these cases, it is important to start with smaller doses and increase slowly without exceeding 10 mg of THC per day. Another option is to reduce the dose of conventional analgesics since the use of cannabis as an adjuvant is strongly associated with a decrease or total replacement of opioid treatment without loss of analgesic effect.[212] Likewise, in epileptic patients, it is recommended to reduce the use of conventional antiepileptic drugs when starting treatment with medical cannabis, as there is already evidence that this induces an increase in the **bioavailability** of clobazam.[213] Some professionals suggest that, when possible, concentrations of clobazam and norclobazam be measured to guide dose adjustment.

On the other hand, the potential interaction with anticoagulant drugs such as warfarin may increase the risk of bleeding.[214,215] At the same time, continuous and long-term exposure to high concentrations of cannabinoids may increase platelet counts,[216] increasing the risk of thrombosis. In both cases, prothrombin testing and/or platelet count should be considered to guide dose adjustments and long-term patient monitoring.

Although there is no evidence of these effects in relation to medicinal use, an association between CBD and increased viral infections has already been established. Thus, the periodic evaluation of the immunological status as well

---

[211] Brown JD. "Potential Adverse Drug Events and Drug – Drug Interactions with Medical and Consumer Cannabidiol (CBD) Use." *J Clin Med.* 2019;8.

[212] Boehnke KF, Scott JR, Litinas E, Sisley S, Williams DA, Clauw DJ. P*ills to Pot: Observational Analyses of Cannabis Substitution Among Medical Cannabis Users With Chronic Pain. J Pain.* 2019 Jul;20(7):830–41.

[213] Geffrey AL, Pollack SF, Bruno PL, Thiele EA. "Drug-drug interaction between clobazam and cannabidiol in children with refractory epilepsy." *Epilepsia.* 2015 Aug;56(8):1246–51.

[214] Brown JD. "Potential Adverse Drug Events and Drug – Drug Interactions with Medical and Consumer Cannabidiol (CBD) Use." *J Clin Med.* 2019;8.

[215] Goyal H, Awad HH, Ghali JK. "Role of cannabis in cardiovascular disorders." *J Thorac Dis.* 2017;9(7):2079–92.

[216] Wani IA, Singh B, Khan MA. "Cannabis Abuse and Hematological Variations to Endorse Severe Health Implications Among Kashmiri Youth." *JOJ Nurse Heal Care.* 2018;8(4).

as the vaccination against common viruses is of special importance in immunosuppressed patients.[217]

---

[217] Thiele EA, Marsh ED, French JA, Mazurkiewicz MB, Benbadis SR, Joshi C, et al. "Cannabidiol in patients with seizures associated with Lennox-Gastaut syndrome (GWPCARE4): a randomised, double-blind, placebo-controlled phase 3 trial." *Lancet*. 2018;391(10125):1085–96.

Side Effects of Cannabis

This chapter takes a closer look at the known side effects of cannabis and provides scientifically-backed insights to understand their occurrence and prevent unwanted effects. The following chart is a summary of the most common side effects of cannabis use:

PHYSICAL	PSYCHOLOGICAL
• Abdominal hyperemesis • Cardiac transient tachycardia • Changes in blood pressure • Dizziness • Hand-eye coordination changes • Mild cough with smoke or vapor • Impaired driving	• Dysphoria • Panic attacks • Paranoia

As prescription drug advertisements remind us, all medicines produce side effects. Sometimes, these side effects are physically unpleasant, and in some cases, side effects can even be fatal. Cannabis, too, has some discomforting side effects, but these are primarily mental or psychological rather than physical. Psychological effects may be dose-related but are often related to the public stigma associated with the plant, whereas physical effects are minor. Interestingly, the dependency risk of cannabis is less than that of coffee.[218] In addition, many studies show there is no adverse effect on IQ.[219] Studies that purport to demonstrate this have been poorly designed and did not properly control important variables such as home environment, parents' rearing skills, traumatic brain injury (TBI), ADD, PTSD, and/or use of other drugs both licit and illicit.

Assessing the body of evidence provided by these studies, it can be stated that cannabis is not associated with severe side effects, and it is generally safe and

---

[218] Phillip J. Hilts, "Negative Addictiveness of Drugs," *New York Times*, Aug. 2, 1994.

[219] Jackson, Nicholas J., Joshua D. Isen, Rubin Khoddam, Daniel Irons, Catherine Tuvblad, William G. Iacono, Matt McGue, Adrian Raine, and Laura A. Baker. "Impact of adolescent marijuana use on intelligence: Results from two longitudinal twin studies." Proceedings of the National Academy of Sciences 113, no. 5 (2016): E500-E508

well tolerated.[220] The most common acute adverse effects are dizziness, vomiting, anxiety (with high doses of THC), neurological symptoms (muscle incoordination, speech disorders, difficulty concentrating, sedation, and sleep), decreased cognitive ability, dry mouth, headache, and tachycardia.

Most of the side effects described are associated with THC.[221] However, many of them, and especially the effects derived from its psychotropic potential, can be avoided by consumption together with CBD.[222,223,224] In addition, it is essential to highlight that, in general, the side effects of THC are dose-dependent and present tolerance, decreasing throughout the treatment.[225] The most effective way to avoid its sudden appearance is to perform a correct dose titration, starting with low doses and increasing them until the symptom improves or the adverse effects appear.[226,227,228]

Physical

The most common physical side effects increased blood pressure, cough, sputum production, and bronchospasm when inhaled.

Blood Pressure (BP)

A 1999 Institute of Medicine report found that can raise or lower BP by 5 mm of mercury (mm Hg). Although the report says its effects are not significant, there are reports of orthostatic hypotension in medical cannabis consumers.

---

[220] Ligresti, A., De Petrocellis, L., & Di Marzo, V. (2016). "From phytocannabinoids to cannabinoid receptors and endocannabinoids: pleiotropic physiological and pathological roles through complex pharmacology." *Physiological Reviews, 96*(4), 1593–1659. https://doi.org/10.1152/physrev.00002.2016

[221] Schultes RE. Random thoughts and queries on the botany of cannabis. In: Joyce CBR, Curry Sh, *The botany and chemistry of Cannabis.* J. & A. Churchill: Londres, 1970.

[222] *History of Cannabis – Chinese medicine.* (n.d.). http://antiquecannabisbook.com/chap2B/China/China.htm/

[223] De França, I. S. X., De Souza, J. A., Baptista, R. S., & De Sousa Britto, V. R. (2008). "Medicina popular: benefícios e malefícios das plantas medicinais." *Revista Brasileira De Enfermagem, 61*(2), 201–208. https://doi.org/10.1590/s0034-71672008000200009

[224] Mackie, K. (2008). "Cannabinoid Receptors: Where They are and What They do." *Journal of Neuroendocrinology, 20*(s1), 10–14. https://doi.org/10.1111/j.1365-2826.2008.01671.x

[225] De França, I. S. X., De Souza, J. A., Baptista, R. S., & De Sousa Britto, V. R. (2008). "Medicina popular: benefícios e malefícios das plantas medicinais." *Revista Brasileira De Enfermagem, 61*(2), 201–208. https://doi.org/10.1590/s0034-71672008000200009

[226] *History of Cannabis – Chinese medicine.* (n.d.). http://antiquecannabisbook.com/chap2B/China/China.htm/

[227] De França, I. S. X., De Souza, J. A., Baptista, R. S., & De Sousa Britto, V. R. (2008). "Medicina popular: benefícios e malefícios das plantas medicinais." *Revista Brasileira De Enfermagem, 61*(2), 201–208. https://doi.org/10.1590/s0034-71672008000200009

[228] Herer J, Meyers J, Cabarga L. "Cannabis Drug Use in 19th Century America," in the emperor wears no clothes. Ah Ha Pub., 1998. http://jackherer.com/emperor-3/

These are isolated incidents and most likely involve high doses of THC. Anecdotally, many middle-aged patients using cannabis experienced blood pressure levels dramatically lowered from previously high and abnormal levels.

Side Effects Due to Smoking

Side effects such as cough, increased sputum production, and/or bronchial irritation may occur from smoking.

Cough	Coughing is by far the most common side effect associated with smoking cannabis. This effect is not from cannabis itself but rather from the route and vehicle of administration. Using other methods of respiratory administration, such as a water pipe (bong) or vaporization device, reduces the amount of bronchial irritation, sputum production, and the incidence of cough. Using sublingual tinctures, edibles, or liquids negates the potential cough problem altogether.
Sputum Production	Increased sputum production and bronchial irritation occur with smoked cannabis. This is according to the research and presentations of Dr. Donald Tashkin of UCLA's David Geffen School of Medicine.[229]
Bronchospasm/ Bronchodilation	While bronchospasm can occur, more importantly, cannabis is a bronchodilator. This is relevant to asthmatic patients. Double-blind experiments conducted by Dr. Tashkin at UCLA using smoked cannabis between 0-2% THC (0 being the placebo) as well as 15 mg synthetic THC administered orally found increases in specific airway conductance (bronchodilation) with both smoked and oral methods. He concluded that the broncho-constriction, which might have been expected in asthmatics following inhalation of particulate matter, was not present.[230] The study concluded that THC was effective in relieving exercise-induced bronchospasm. This bronchodilatory action lasted from four to twelve hours after administration. In 1977, the same UCLA team used aerosolized THC in 5 mg and 20 mg doses. All doses produced similar, significant bronchodilation. The lower dose produced fewer physical (tachycardia) or psychological (high) side effects than the higher dose of smoked cannabis.[231]

---

[229] Tashkin, Donald P. "Effects of marijuana smoking on the lung." *Annals of the American Thoracic Society* 10, no. 3 (2013): 239-247.

[230] Gong, Henry, Donald P. Tashkin, Michael S. Simmons, Barry Calvarese, and Bertrand J. Shapiro. "Acute and subacute bronchial effects of oral cannabinoids." *Clinical Pharmacology & Therapeutics* 35, no. 1 (1984): 26-32.

[231] Tashkin, Donald P., Sheldon Reiss, Bertrand J. Shapiro, Barry Calvarese, James L. Olsen, and Jon W. Lodge. "Bronchial effects of aerosolized ?9-tetrahydrocannabinol in healthy and asthmatic subjects." *American Review of Respiratory Disease* 115, no. 1 (1977): 57-65.

Does Cannabis Cause Lung Cancer?

Smoking cannabis has been associated with assorted respiratory symptoms, increased risk of bronchitis, increased cough, sputum production, and bronchial irritation. The suspicion was that cannabis smoking might increase cancer risk, which was only heightened because smoked cannabis does contain carcinogens and is a bronchial irritant. But does cannabis cause lung cancer? The short answer is no; it does not increase the risk of getting lung cancer.

> *Studies indicate that, due to the antiproliferative effect of cannabinoids, cannabis smokers are at a lower risk of developing lung cancer than non-smokers.*[232]

As evidence has mounted about the medicinal uses of cannabis, the government has tried to shift its argument for maintaining the Schedule I status from "cannabis is very bad" to "smoking anything is bad." While it sounds reasonable, it turns out that the idea that smoking cannabis causes lung cancer ignores the epidemiology and the science.

Cannabis smoke, unlike tobacco, has never been shown to cause lung cancer. In fact, because of the antiproliferative effect of cannabinoids and terpenes, studies indicate that among cannabis users, there is a lower risk of lung cancer than non-smokers. Several mechanisms contribute to cannabis's anti-proliferative effect, including inhibiting angiogenic growth factor (AGF), which is emitted by cancer cells while trying to develop their own blood vessels. Additionally, cannabis causes apoptosis in cancer cells.

This lung cancer issue was definitively answered by the 2004 National Institute on Drug Abuse (NIDA) funded 2,100-subject study by respected UCLA pulmonology researcher Dr. Donald P. Tashkin. He found that cannabis smokers showed statistically lower cancer rates than non-smokers (i.e., people who smoked nothing at all). Even heavy cannabis smoking did not increase the risk of lung cancer. Tashkin concluded that cannabis smoking—"even heavy long-term use"—does not cause cancer of the lung, upper airways, or esophagus.[233]

This conclusion is especially significant because Tashkin had long believed in

---

[232] Werner, C. (2011). *Marijuana: Gateway to health: How cannabis protects us from cancer and Alzheimers disease.* San Francisco: Dachstar Press.

[233] Kaufman, Marc. "Study finds no cancer-marijuana connection." *The Washington Post* 26 (2006).

the likelihood of a causal relationship between cannabis and lung cancer. This was because of the presence of several carcinogens contained in cannabis smoke and the proven bronchial irritation associated with smoking cannabis. Tashkin's results upset NIDA, and although he had previously received numerous NIDA grants, NIDA worked hard to bury or misrepresent the results of his study.

Cardiovascular Effects

A 2002 article by R.T. Jones entitled "Cardiovascular System Effects of Marijuana" points out that tolerance to cardiac effects is rapid. The author states, "With repeated exposure, supine blood pressure decreases slightly, orthostatic hypotension disappears, blood volume increases, heart rate slows, and circulatory responses to exercise and Valsalva maneuver are diminished."[234]

Positive Cardiovascular Effects

There are positive cardiovascular effects of cannabis. It helps minimize cell death in an ischemic event. Inflammation has been found to play a central role in vascular occlusions from atrioventricular septal defects. Cannabis is an anti-inflammatory. Animal research has shown cannabinoids can decrease cardiac damage caused by transient decreased blood flow (e.g., cardiac ischemia).[235]

The beneficial cardiac potential for CBD was one of several anti-inflammatory constituents highlighted in a 2013 review published in *The Journal of Pharmacology*. The review explains that in rodent models, cannabis reduced vascular tension, a condition that causes additional strain on the heart. Cannabis has also been shown to protect the arteries from glucose damage. The same article stated that cannabis reduces general inflammation in blood vessels.[236]

The several active constituents in cannabis engage with the cardiac system to produce protective effects. A rodent study published in *The International Journal of Cardiology* found that ECS deficiencies could contribute to chronic

---

[234] Jones, Reese T. "Cardiovascular system effects of marijuana." *The Journal of Clinical Pharmacology* 42, no. S1 (2002).

[235] Mendizábal VE, Adler-Graschinsky E. "Cannabinoids as therapeutic agents in cardiovascular disease: a tale of passions and illusions." *Br J Pharmacol*. 2007;151(4):427–440. doi:10.1038/sj.bjp.0707261

[236] Stanley, Christopher P., William H. Hind, and Saoirse E. O'sullivan. "Is the cardiovascular system a therapeutic target for cannabidiol?" B*ritish Journal of Clinical Pharmacology* 75, no. 2 (2013): 313-322.

ASHD (atherosclerotic heart disease). Mice that had lower levels of cannabinoid receptors (CB1) suffered more heart abnormalities than mice with healthy CB1 expression. Researchers "found that CB1 deficiency contributed to the extensive chronic cardiac remodeling...revealing a new role of CB1 in [chronic heart failure]."[237]

CB2 receptor activation is anti-atherogenic, meaning it impedes the development of fatty plaque in the arteries. Steffens et al. showed a decrease in the progression of atherosclerotic lesions in murine models after oral administration of low-dose THC.[238] THC also downregulates Th1 immune response cells, the primary cells in atherosclerotic lesions. A synthetic CB2 receptor agonist was shown to decrease the size of plaque and macrophage content in atherosclerotic lesions. The CB2 receptor agonist also reduced oxidized-LDL-mediated NF-kb activation and pro-inflammatory cytokine expression.

A 15-year longitudinal follow-up of 3,617 adults in the Coronary Artery Risk Development in Young Adults (CARDYA) study found there was no association between cannabis use and cardiovascular risk after adjusting for confounding factors.[239]

Cannabis Hyperemesis Syndrome (CHS)

Cannabis hyperemesis syndrome (CHS) was, until recently, considered a relatively rare condition of excessive and severe bouts of vomiting with high doses of THC. With the advent of adult use legalization, CHS has become more common. It usually occurs in daily long-term users of cannabis, but it can also occur with a single high dose consumption.

The mechanism is still unknown. It may be that, like some other therapeutic substances, a small amount of a substance effectively treats a symptom while a large dose can cause the very same symptom, in this case, nausea and vomiting. It still isn't clear why some heavy users get the syndrome and others don't.

---

[237] Liao, Yulin, Jianping Bin, Tao Luo, Hui Zhao, Catherine Ledent, Masanori Asakura, Dingli Xu, Seiji Takashima, and Masafumi Kitakaze. "CB1 cannabinoid receptor deficiency promotes cardiac remodeling induced by pressure overload in mice." *International Journal of Cardiology* 167, no. 5 (2013): 1936-1944.

[238] Steffens, Sabine, Niels R. Veillard, Claire Arnaud, Graziano Pelli, Fabienne Burger, Christian Staub, Andreas Zimmer, Jean-Louis Frossard, and François Mach. "Low dose oral cannabinoid therapy reduces progression of atherosclerosis in mice." *Nature* 434, no. 7034 (2005): 782.

[239] Rodondi, Nicolas, Mark James Pletcher, Kiang Liu, Stephen Benjamin Hulley, and Stephen Sidney. "Marijuana use, diet, body mass index, and cardiovascular risk factors (from the CARDIA study)." *American Journal of Cardiology* 98, no. 4 (2006): 478-484.

Hyperemesis in heavy users can be alarming because it may last for hours or days. This is unlike excessive vomiting from a one-time large dose. These are three phases: the prodromal phase, the hyperemetic phase, and the recovery phase.

- **Prodromal phase**: The main symptoms are often early morning nausea and abdominal pain. Some people use more cannabis because they think it will help stop the nausea. In rare cases, this phase may last for several days.
- **Hyperemetic phase**: Symptoms during this time may include ongoing nausea, repeated episodes of vomiting, and abdominal pain. This is associated with decreased food intake, weight loss, and fluid loss (dehydration). Many people take hot showers during the day to ease their nausea. That may be because of how the hot temperature affects the hypothalamus, which affects both temperature regulation and vomiting.
- **Recovery phase**: During this phase, symptoms go away, and normal eating is possible again. This phase can last days or weeks, or in some instances, until the person tries cannabis again.

Psychological

The most common unwanted psychological effect is dysphoria.

When a person is "high," they recognize it and adjust their dose accordingly. While there are many beneficial psychological effects to cannabis, there are some psychological side effects that may occur. These include paranoia, panic attacks (usually high-THC use in inexperienced users), and impaired judgment.

Dysphoria

Dysphoria is excessive, unpleasant euphoria. Dysphoria is usually related to inexperienced users consuming too much THC and not enough CBD. Dysphoria is more likely to occur when administered orally but can also occur with smoking. On the other hand, euphoria itself can be therapeutic. Dr. Donald Abrams, UCSF Medical School professor, oncologist, and AIDS treatment researcher, says, "In my patient population, a little euphoria is a good thing."[240]

In *New York Times* columnist Maureen Dowd's 2014 article "Don't Harsh Our Mellow, Dude,"[241] she offers an excellent example of the adverse effect of an inexperienced user consuming a high dose of an edible THC product. It appears Dowd did not understand that cannabis, much like most medication consumed by the oral route of administration, takes 45-75 minutes to take effect. She was impatient. After taking two 10 mg pieces of chocolate, she ate the whole 100 mg bar. In response, the June 20, 2014 issue of *The Week* put it this way, "Dowd ate too much of a weed-laced candy bar, which had no dosing instructions, and spent eight hours curled up in a paranoid, catatonic, hallucinatory state."[242]

This is not a surprise. Dowd had not thoroughly researched her subject, so rather than using the respiratory route of administration where she could have more easily self-titrated the dose she would consume, she orally consumed too much of a high-THC chocolate bar (edible). Dowd was unaware that the effects were not immediate and could last up to several hours. Therefore, for an inexperienced user, inhalation is the preferable route, at least until the proper oral dose is found.

Treating Dysphoria

Whether smoking a high-THC cannabis cultivar for the first time or eating a high-potency THC product, getting "too stoned" (dysphoria) is something that happens to many people.

Both THC and CBD dosage affect a cannabis consumer's experience. Beginners are most susceptible to dysphoria. While this can be uncomfortable, it is not a life-threatening or permanent problem. Here are some common approaches:

---

[240] "The Science Behind Medical Marijuana: An Interview with Donald Abrams." HealthTalk Live. Last Modified February 2008. https://www.everydayhealth.com/healthy-living/webcasts/the-science-behind-medical-marijuana.aspx/.

[241] Dowd, Maureen. 2014. "Opinion | Don't Harsh Our Mellow, Dude." *The New York Times*, June 4, 2014, sec. Opinion. https://www.nytimes.com/2014/06/04/opinion/dowd-dont-harsh-our-mellow-dude.html.

[242] "Preventing Reefer Madness." The Week. Last Modified June 20, 2014. http://www.antarcticajournal.com/preventing-reefer-madness/.

Titrating THC doses, especially with ingested cannabis
- Start with a low dose (~2.5 mg) of full spectrum THC extract.

CBD
- Increase the CBD dose, unless treating pain, where a higher CBD to THC ratio (greater than 1:1) can interfere with analgesia. CBD blocks the euphoria associated with cannabis.

Other valuable substances besides CBD
- **Terpenes** (citrus, black pepper, pine): Limonene, beta-caryophyllene, and pinene help to lessen the anxiety associated with cannabis use. Limonene is found in citrus fruits like oranges, lemons, limes, and grapefruit. Squeezing fresh juice into water with freshly cracked beta-caryophyllene-rich black pepper may help mitigate anxious or paranoid feelings. Eating pistachios or pine nuts, both high in the terpene pinene, may also lessen anxiety.
- **Ibuprofen**: Research indicates that ibuprofen may counteract some effects of THC, especially when it comes to memory and mental acuity.
- **Citicoline:** Citicoline is used to treat victims of head trauma and neurodegenerative disorders. Citicoline blocks the effect of THC-induced euphoria or dysphoria, and its effects are accelerated when taken with citrus.

Other non-pharmacological actions
- **Use suppository route of administration:** Suppositories are usually paraffin-infused with a therapeutic substance. The medication is absorbed through the rectum by three separate veins: the lower, middle, and upper rectal veins. The lower and middle rectal veins drain directly into the general circulation, while the upper drains into the portal vein, which flows to the liver. This means that much of the THC is deposited in the body's adipose tissue and interstitial fluid rather than going directly to the liver, where THC is metabolized into the highly psychotropic 11-hydroxy-THC.
- **Bathe or shower**
- **Hydrate**
- **Eat**
- **Exercise/movement**

IQ Not Affected

In a first-of-its-kind study, scientists analyzed long-term cannabis users by comparing identical twins. Researchers compared IQ changes in twin siblings who either used or abstained from cannabis for ten years. After taking environmental factors into account, in over 3,000 individuals, *the scientists found no measurable link between cannabis use and lower IQ.*[243] This number is in contrast to the much smaller studies that report a negative correlation between cannabis smoking and IQ levels.[244,245] The combined participant size in these studies was less than 125 individuals.

"This is a very well-conducted study... and a welcome addition to the literature," says Valerie Curran, a psycho-pharmacologist at the University College London. She and her colleagues reached "broadly the same conclusions" in a separate, non-twin study of more than 2,000 British teenagers.[246]

Pregnancy

The effect of maternal cannabis use on the developing fetus during pregnancy is controversial. However, the idea that THC is deleterious to the developing mind has never been proven to be a fact. The American College of Obstetricians and Gynecologists recommends that pregnant or breast-feeding women—and women considering pregnancy—should be screened for and discouraged from using cannabis and other substances. However, there is not a gold standard study demonstrating significant adverse effects. Other studies show no effect on the fetus, and some offer a benefit.

One of the first documented uses of cannabis in female reproduction was within the Egyptian civilization around 2350 BCE, and research points to interactions between female reproduction and the endocannabinoid system. The endocannabinoid system is responsible for neuronal development. Embryonic implantation requires anandamide, an endocannabinoid that protects the developing brain from naturally occurring trauma-induced neuronal loss. Interestingly, suckling initiation in the newborn is stimulated

---

[243] Jackson, Nicholas J., Joshua D. Isen, Rubin Khoddam, Daniel Irons, Catherine Tuvblad, William G. Iacono, Matt McGue, Adrian Raine, and Laura A. Baker. "Impact of adolescent marijuana use on intelligence: Results from two longitudinal twin studies." Proceedings of the National Academy of Sciences 113, no. 5 (2016): E500-E508.

[244] Lyons, Michael J., J. L. Bar, M. S. Panizzon, R. Toomey, S. Eisen, H. Xian, and M. T. Tsuang. "Neuropsychological consequences of regular marijuana use: a twin study." *Psychological Medicine* 34, no. 7 (2004): 1239-1250.

[245] Fried, Peter, Barbara Watkinson, Deborah James, and Robert Gray. "Current and former marijuana use: preliminary findings of a longitudinal study of effects on IQ in young adults." *Canadian Medical Association Journal* 166, no. 7 (2002): 887-891.

[246] Underwood, Emily. "Twins Study Finds No Evidence that Marijuana Lowers IQ in Teens." *Science Magazine*. January 18, 2016. http://www.sciencemag.org/news/2016/01/twins-study-finds-no-evidence-marijuana-lowers-iq-teens

by activation of the CB1 receptors in the neonatal brain.[247]

Ciara A. Torres, PhD, of Columbia University, reviewed over 30 studies on prenatal use of cannabis. Most of the studies were funded by the National Institute on Drug Abuse (NIDA). Of over 380 variables, only eight of the variables in these studies were abnormal or negative, but there was no consistency in these negative findings. Furthermore, many of the results were positive, but the findings were obscured because the write-ups, according to Dr. Torres, were slanted to reporting what researchers seemed to think the funding source wanted to hear.[248]

Due to the problems caused by confounding factors and routine lack of control of these factors (nutrition, environment, other drug use), it cannot be said with certainty that cannabis has any adverse effects on the developing fetus. However, it also can be noted that no unequivocal compelling scientific or epidemiologic evidence demonstrates it. As with the ingestion of any therapeutic agent during pregnancy, cannabis should be used with caution.

NIDA Study in Jamaica

Melody Dreher, RN, PhD, did a series of NIDA-funded studies in Jamaica in 1968 and 1973. Dr. Dreher compared children of women who had used cannabis during pregnancy against children of women who had not. Dr. Dreher's study demonstrated no problems for children whose mothers used cannabis during pregnancy and showed that these children actually performed better in school and met developmental landmarks sooner than children of non-cannabis-using mothers. Her study, therefore, found that there were no adverse effects on the child if a mother had used cannabis during pregnancy and/or while breastfeeding.[249]

Dr. Dreher used the Brazelton Neonatal Behavioral Assessment Scale to compare the babies of 24 Jamaican women who had used ganja (cannabis) with a control group. At one month, the children of the cannabis users had better scores than the non-cannabis users, which the researchers attributed

---

[247] Wilson-King, G. (2019). "Thirteenth National Clinical Conference on Cannabis Therapeutics." Tampa Bay, April 11-13, 2019

[248] "ACOG Committee Opinion". *The American College of Obstetricians and Gynecologists*. Last Modified October 2017. https://www.acog.org/Clinical-Guidance-and-Publications/Committee-Opinions/Committee-on-Obstetric-Practice/Marijuana-Use-During-Pregnancy-and-Lactation

[249] Torres, Ciara A., and Carl L. Hart. "Prenatal cannabis exposure and cognitive functioning: A critical review." *Drug & Alcohol Dependence* 171 (2017): e204.

to "the cultural positioning and social and economic characteristics of mothers using marijuana that select for the use of cannabis but also promote neonatal development."

Dr. Dreher did ethnographic studies that examined the lifestyles of mothers who used ganja and mothers who did not and compared behavioral characteristics of neonates from both groups in the first month of life. She and her research team returned five years later and did a follow-up study on the children.

Her studies are among the few that have measured how much ganja mothers consumed. Dr. Dreher noted that she "wasn't sitting in a clinic somewhere divorced from women's lives asking them how much marijuana they'd used."[250] Her research team was in a community and the field where they observed these women and checked out their reports. Her team knew the type, potency, and how much ganja the women were consuming.

When NIDA saw that the results were favorable to cannabis, they ceased funding the study. The overwhelming consensus in the cannabinoid medicine community, however, is that the research findings of Dr. Dreher were profound and far-reaching.

Other Studies and Their Findings

- No difference in birth weight, shorter birth length, smaller head circumference[251]
- Drs. John P. Morgan and Lynn Zimmer assert, "Marijuana has no reliable impact on birth size, length of gestation... or the occurrence of physical abnormalities."[252]
- A 1999 study in Copenhagen concluded that "the use of cannabis is not a major prognostic factor regarding the outcome of pregnancy."[253]

---

[250] Dreher, Melanie C., Kevin Nugent, and Rebekah Hudgins. "Prenatal marijuana exposure and neonatal outcomes in Jamaica: an ethnographic study." *Pediatrics* 93, no. 2 (1994): 254-260.

[251] Fergusson, David M., L. John Horwood, and Kate Northstone. "Maternal use of cannabis and pregnancy outcome." *BJOG: An International Journal of Obstetrics & Gynecology* 109, no. 1 (2002): 21-27.

[252] Morgan, John P., and Lynn Zimmer. "Exposing marijuana myths: A review of the scientific evidence." *Cannabis Science/Cannabis* Wissenschaft. Frankfurt Am Main: Peter Lang Verlag (1997): 101-126.

[253] Balle, J., M. J. Olofsson, and J. Hilden. "Cannabis and pregnancy." *Ugeskr Laeger* 161, no. 36 (1999): 5024-8

- A 2002 survey of 12,060 British women did not demonstrate significant differences in growth among newborns exposed to cannabis in utero versus those with no exposure when controlling for confounding factors such as the mother's age, pre-pregnancy weight, and the self-reported use of tobacco, alcohol, caffeine and/or cocaine after controlling for maternal tobacco usage.[254]
- A 1997 Australian study of 32,483 mothers also reported, "There is inadequate evidence that cannabis, at the amount typically consumed by pregnant women, causes low birth weight."[255]
- More recently, a large-scale case-control study published in the *Journal Pediatric and Perinatal Epidemiology* determined that mothers who reported using cannabis during pregnancy suffered no increased risk of bearing children with acute myeloid leukemia, a cancer known to occur in adolescents under age 15.[256]

Research into the short-term effects of prenatal cannabis exposure has mixed or inconclusive results on birth outcomes:

PURPORTED EFFECT	EVIDENCE
Preterm delivery	Mixed evidence
Low birth weight/SGA	Mixed evidence
Fetal growth	Mixed evidence
Withdrawal	Mixed evidence

Limitations of Studies

Because of limitations, the studies done to address this issue are not gold-standard double-blind studies. The fact is that it is much easier to do studies on mice than it is on humans because there are many confounding factors.

---

[254] Fergusson, David M., L. John Horwood, and Kate Northstone. "Maternal use of cannabis and pregnancy outcome." *BJOG: An International Journal of Obstetrics & Gynecology* 109, no. 1 (2002): 21-27.

[255] English, D. R., G. K. Hulse, E. Milne, C. D. J. Holman, and C. I. Bower. "Maternal cannabis use and birth weight: a meta-analysis." *Addiction* 92, no. 11 (1997): 1553-1560. 121

[256] Trivers, Katrina F., Ann C. Mertens, Julie A. Ross, Michael Steinbuch, Andrew F. Olshan, and Leslie L. Robison. "Parental marijuana use and risk of childhood acute myeloid leukemia: a report from the Children's Cancer Group (United States and Canada)." *Pediatric and Perinatal Epidemiology* 20, no. 2 (2006): 110-118.

These confounding factors include, but are not limited to:

- Environmental risk factors
- Family history
- Maternal IQ/cognitive ability
- Socioeconomic status
- Recruitment methods
- Assessment measures
- Medical issues (PTSD, ADD, TBI)
- Drug use (alcohol, tobacco, cocaine, heroin, prescription)

Conclusion Regarding Prenatal Exposure to Cannabinoids

Cannabis does not have any well-documented adverse impact on a developing fetus. Dr. Dreher's work from Jamaica examined the birth weights and early development of babies exposed to cannabis compared to non-exposed infants. Mothers in the study reported that they occasionally mixed cannabis with tea as an alternative to smoking. Her study reported no significant physical or psychological differences in three-day-old newborns of heavy cannabis-using mothers and found that exposed children performed better on a variety of physiological and autonomic tests than non-exposed children at 30 days of life. However, this latter trend was suggested to have been a result of the socio-economic status of the mothers rather than a result of prenatal cannabis exposure.

Conventional wisdom says that pregnant women should avoid any drug or food that is not needed. This would include alcohol, tobacco, prescription drugs, food additives, preservatives, coffee, and tea, as well as cannabis. However, cannabis helps treat nausea and anxiety as well as stimulate appetite, so there may be an argument for continued use of cannabis during pregnancy in some cases.

Dependence

Though scientific evidence has proven cannabis dependency to be real, this dependency has been overhyped, overplayed, and exaggerated. The dependency risk associated with cannabis is, in fact, less than that of coffee. In 1953, Thompson and Proctor summed up the attitude of the great majority of the medical profession, stating, "The use of cannabis does not give rise to biological or physiological dependence and discontinuance of the drug does not result in withdrawal symptoms."[257]

In 1976, Stephen Szara of the National Institute on Drug Abuse (NIDA) categorically stated, "The question of physical dependence... has been answered with a flat no. No physical dependence of the type seen in opiates has been seen in man, and this is true even today."[258] It is easier to stop using cannabis than it is to stop drinking coffee or smoking nicotine-containing substances.

In 1999, the Institute of Medicine (IOM) concluded, "Experimental animals that are given the opportunity to self-administer cannabinoids generally do not choose to do so, which has led to the conclusion that they (e.g., cannabinoids) are not reinforcing or rewarding." The IOM report states there is a very low incidence of cannabis "dependence." They reasoned, "Millions of Americans have tried marijuana, but most are not regular users...[and] few marijuana users become dependent on it."[259]

Most cannabis users without a chronic or fatal illness voluntarily cease their cannabis smoking by their late 20s or early 30s, often citing health or professional concerns and/or the decision to start a family. Contrast this pattern with that of the typical tobacco smoker, many of whom start as teens and continue smoking daily for the rest of their lives.

Dependency Risk is Comparable to Coffee

When the dependency risk for cannabis is compared to other substances, including coffee, cannabis is considered by experts to have the lowest dependency risk. A 1994 *New York Times* article backed this claim by citing

---

[257] Grivas, Kleanthis, and Deborah Whitehouse. *Cannabis: Marihuana-Hashish*. Minerva Press, 1997.

[258] *Ibid.*

[259] Joy, Janet, Stanley J. Watson, Jr., and John A. Benson, eds. *Marijuana and Medicine: Assessing the Science Base*. Washington D.C.: National Academy Press, 1999.

work by Dr. Jack Henningfield, then with NIDA, and Dr. Neal Benowitz of the University of California at San Francisco. Henningfield and Benowitz rated the addictive symptoms of cannabis against other commonly used drugs, including heroin, alcohol, nicotine, coffee, and cocaine. Overall, "Marijuana was ranked lowest for withdrawal symptoms, tolerance, and dependence (addiction) potential; it ranked close to caffeine in the degree of reinforcement and higher than caffeine and nicotine only in the degree of intoxication." It has also been reported that "Even in cases of high daily intake, such as the 94-day study of high dose cannabis, with its sudden cessation; withdrawal symptoms were transient and mild."[260] In fact, the authors of the aforementioned report found less than 10% of marijuana users ever exhibited symptoms of dependence as defined by the American Psychiatric Association's DSM-3 criteria. By comparison, 15% of alcohol users, 17% of cocaine users, and a whopping 32% of cigarette smokers statistically exhibited symptoms of drug dependence.[261,262]

Mild Withdrawal Symptoms

Reese Jones, MD, a critic of medical cannabis, designed a study aiming to demonstrate withdrawal symptoms from THC. He placed volunteers on 210 mg of dronabinol (synthetic THC) a day for 20 days. This medicine, containing only THC, has none of the hundreds of other naturally occurring plant molecules (such as CBD) that would help mitigate the effects of THC-induced euphoria. This study's daily dose is equivalent to smoking 20-40 joints of botanical cannabis per day. At the end of 20 days, the THC was stopped abruptly. This is a formula calculated to maximize any drug withdrawal symptoms that might occur. He found only mild withdrawal symptoms in individuals taking the high doses of synthetic Δ^9-THC under laboratory conditions.

The 210 mg per day that Dr. Jones's subjects were given is 15–30 times higher than what would be ingested by the average consumer. Benowitz and Jones reported initial tachycardia and hypertension in volunteer subjects. These effects were short-lived as they found tolerance developed to tachycardia and the central nervous system effects over the 20-day experiment. In general, participants' blood pressure reduced and stabilized at around 95/65

---

[260] Lambert, Didier M., ed. *Cannabinoids in Nature and Medicine*. John Wiley & Sons, 2009.

[261] *Ibid.*

[262] Wiese, B. M. (2019). *Thirteenth National Clinical Conference on Cannabis Therapeutics*. Tampa Bay, April 11-13, 2019

mm Hg.[263]

Substance Dependency

Substance dependency is defined as using a substance in such a manner that the consumption of that substance interferes with important aspects of a person's life, be it financial, occupational, educational, recreational, social, familial, or other important parts of life. There certainly is a condition of drug dependency with cannabis. It can be a symptom of some underlying conditions, such as anxiety, PTSD, and/or depression. If present, these conditions must be addressed. Treating drug dependency as an isolated condition without treating the underlying cause is a recipe for treatment failure. On the other hand, addressing the motivation for excessive and or inappropriate substance use can be helpful in promoting a successful outcome.

Cannabis Abuse Disorder

Psychiatric diagnoses are categorized by the American Psychiatric Association (APA) in their Diagnostic and Statistical Manual of Mental Disorders (DSM-5). DSM-5 covers all mental health disorders for both children and adults. In the 5th and newest edition, the APA has redefined its section on cannabis. The DSM-5 lists "cannabis use disorder." The definition is only somewhat different than for "cannabis abuse" that appeared in the previous edition of this manual, the DSM-4.

The DSM-5 defines use disorder as "A problematic pattern of cannabis use leading to clinically significant impairment or distress, as manifested by at least two of the following, occurring within a 12-month period:[264]

- Cannabis is often taken in larger amounts or over a longer period than was intended.
- There is a persistent desire or unsuccessful efforts to cut down or control cannabis use.
- A great deal of time is spent in activities necessary to obtain cannabis, use cannabis, or recover from its effects.

---

[263] Jones, Reese T., Neal L. Benowitz and Ronald I. Herning. "Clinical relevance of cannabis tolerance and dependence." *The Journal of Clinical Pharmacology* 21, no. S1 (1981).

[264] *Diagnostic and Statistical Manual of Mental Disorders*, 5th Edition. American Psychiatric Association, 2013.

- Craving, or a strong desire or urge to use cannabis.
- Recurrent cannabis use resulting in a failure to fulfill major role obligations at work, school, or home.
- Continued cannabis use despite having persistent or recurrent social or interpersonal problems caused or exacerbated by the effects of cannabis.
- Important social, occupational, or recreational activities are given up or reduced because of cannabis use.
- Recurrent cannabis use in situations in which it is physically hazardous. (Note: the FDA says THC may be used while doing dangerous activities if it does not interfere with those activities.)
- Cannabis use is continued despite knowledge of having a persistent or recurrent physical or psychological problem that is likely to have been caused or exacerbated by cannabis.
- Tolerance, as defined by either a (1) need for markedly increased cannabis dose to achieve intoxication or a desired effect of (2) markedly diminished effect with continued use of the same amount of the substance.[265]
- Withdrawal, per the DSM-5's withdrawal, is the characteristic withdrawal syndrome for cannabis, or cannabis is taken to relieve or avoid withdrawal symptoms. (Note: in clinical practice, withdrawal symptoms are generally mild and relatively rare.)
- Cannabis is taken to relieve or avoid withdrawal symptoms."[266]

Considerations

In order to focus treatment resources on those with substance abuse issues, it is important to distinguish use from abuse. Few would argue with assisting and treating someone whose life is problematic and drug abuse has been a contributing factor. Such abuse occurs infrequently and is rarely seen in the medical use of cannabis. Most people who are prescribed or recommended therapeutic use of psychotropic drugs such as Marinol and Cesamet take them appropriately with the same or fewer side effects than many other categories of drugs. This is certainly true of the low side-effect profile of

---

[265] Feinberg, I., Jones, R., Walker, J. M., Cavness, C., & March, J. (2016, January 4). "Effects of high dosage delta-9-tetrahydrocannabinol on sleep patterns in man." Retrieved from https://ascpt.onlinelibrary.wiley.com/doi/abs/10.1002/cpt1975174458

[266] *Diagnostic and Statistical Manual of Mental Disorders*, 5th Edition. American Psychiatric Association, 2013.

cannabis.[267]

While there is no doubt that there is something that can be identified as cannabis dependence (relying too heavily on cannabis to deal with problems of the day), there is no such thing as a classical addiction to cannabis.

---

[267] "Your Government is Lying to You (Again) About Marijuana." *NORML* http://norml.org/library/item/your-government-is-lying-to-you-again-about-marijuana

Toxicology

Toxicology refers to drug testing to measure THC in a person's blood, urine, or hair. It is important to remember that a toxicology *result* shows the presence or absence of a drug or its principal metabolite and is not by itself evidence of substance abuse. A toxicology test does not distinguish use from abuse, nor does it indicate the nature and reason for that substance use. As with most conditions, history is a critical element of any diagnosis.

From applicable regulations, it is clear that it is okay for patients to receive THC in the form of the prescription Marinol but not if it comes in the cannabis plant, which contains hundreds of different cannabinoids, terpenes, flavonoids, and phenols. Blood, hair, and urine analysis tests used by commercial laboratories to detect cannabis are not a test for cannabis but a test for THC and two of its principal metabolites, 9-carboxy-THC and 11-hydroxy-THC. The reasoning here is that the toxicology screen is looking for the presence of illicit drugs, not licit drugs.

Medical review officers (MROs), the physicians responsible for interpreting the results of employee urinalysis, use toxicology interpretation guidelines, a little-noted but significant fact. These guidelines instruct the MROs to report those testing positive for THC as negative if the subject is being legally prescribed THC (dronabinol). This guideline treats synthetic THC the same as one would any other prescribed medication. For instance, a positive for hydrocodone in a patient prescribed Norco, which contains hydrocodone, would be reported as a negative.[268]

Thus, per the Medical Review Officers Association guidelines, it is okay if a urine or blood toxicology test is positive for THC and/or its metabolites as a result of prescription Marinol. A separate test to rule out cannabis as the source of THC is an additional expense and is rarely done.

The presence of THC and its metabolites in the blood doesn't indicate impairment; it suggests that cannabis was consumed sometime in the last four to seven days.

---

[268] "Medical Review Officers." US Department of Transportation. https://www.transportation.gov/odapc/mro/.

Cannabis Use and Driving

The National Highway Traffic Safety Administration's (NHTSA) online factsheet states, "It is difficult to establish a relationship between a person's THC blood or plasma concentration and performance impairing effects... It is inadvisable to try and predict effects based on blood THC concentrations alone, and currently impossible to predict specific effects based on THC COOH [carbolic acid] concentrations."[269] The NHTSA found no increased risk of auto accidents from the use of cannabis and stated that cannabis may lead to slower, more careful driving.

The Food and Drug Administration (FDA) Warning

The FDA is unconcerned about THC levels and driving and does not believe that the mere presence of THC or its metabolites in a patient's bloodstream is an absolute contraindication to driving, operating heavy equipment, or engaging in dangerous activity. The FDA warning is a clear and very significant statement:

> WARNING: Patients receiving treatment with MARINOL® Capsules should be specifically warned not to drive, operate machinery, or engage in any hazardous activity until it is established that they are able to tolerate the drug and to perform such tasks safely.[270]

The FDA-approved warning clearly states that it is permissible to drive, operate heavy equipment, or engage in dangerous activities so long as the use of THC (dronabinol) does not interfere with those activities. So, according to the FDA, it is permissible to drive a motor vehicle without reference to blood THC levels.

Many physicians put some form of this FDA warning on their recommendation for medical cannabis. This phrase might be added, "Don't drive if you are and/or feel impaired." If a medicinal cannabis patient gets in a severe accident and can be proven to be impaired, the legal risks and consequences can be devastating. Ensure the patient is aware that they should take the FDA warning seriously.

---

[269] "Cannabis/Marijuana (Δ-9-Tetrahydrocannabinol, THC)." National Highway Traffic Safety Administration. https://www.nhtsa.gov/sites/nhtsa.dot.gov/files/documents/812440-marijuana-impaired-driving-report-to-congress.pdf

[270] Ibid.

While many patients do not feel that the medicinal use of cannabis impairs their driving, others think it may or does and refrain from medicating until they are finished driving for the day. Even if a patient is not impaired, many jurisdictions are quick to charge the patient if the odor of cannabis is in the car, on the patient's clothing, or if there is cannabis or drug paraphernalia somewhere in the car. Drivers must use the same common sense as they would with prescription drugs and alcohol.

Some people find it difficult to process this FDA conclusion. Part of the difficulty in accepting it is that this requires recognizing the fact that alcohol differs from most other psychoactive substances. It does not bind to specific receptors. It is a non-specific neural depressant.

In 2014, the NHTSA stated, "The alcohol laws are based on evidence concerning the decreased ability of drivers across the population to function safely at these [blood alcohol content levels]...Such evidence is not currently available for concentrations of other drugs."[271] Most medications, including cannabinoids, act by affecting specific receptors. Also, considerable human variability exists, so some people have more side effects than others.

Measuring Impairment

The US Department of Transportation (DOT) has stated, "It is not possible to conclude anything about a driver's impairment on the basis of his/her plasma concentrations of THC and THC-COOH determined in a single sample."[272]

Tolerance contributes to the conclusion in the February 2015 and 1993 NHTSA reports, underscoring an important point: "The measurable presence of THC in a person's system doesn't correlate with impairment in the same way that alcohol concentration does."

The 2015 NHTSA report was very clear: "At the current time, specific drug concentration levels cannot be reliably equated with a specific degree of driver impairment."[273] Little appears to have changed from the National

---

[271] National Highway Traffic Safety Administration. Op. cit.

[272] "Marijuana and Actual Driving Performance, Effects of THC on Driving Performance," US Department of Transportation, NHTSA, November 1993. http://druglibrary.org/schaffer/misc/driving/dot78_1.htm/.

[273] Ingraham, Christopher. "Stone Drivers are a lot safer than drunk ones, new federal data show." *The Washington Post*. February 9, 2015. https://www.washingtonpost.com/news/wonk/wp/2015/02/09/stoned-drivers-are-a-lot-safer-than-drunk-ones-new-federal-data-show/?utm_term=.f7f307bb0840/.

Highway Traffic Administration 1993 Safety Study Report, which stated, "THC's adverse effects on driving performance appear relatively small," and "Evidence from the present and previous studies strongly suggests that alcohol encourages risky driving, whereas THC encourages greater caution."[274]

An article by C.T. Lamers stated, "Performance as rated on the Driving Proficiency Scale did not differ between treatments (cannabis versus placebo). It was concluded that the effects of low doses of THC...on visual search and general driving proficiency are minimal." Using driving instructors' performance scores, Lamers and Ramaekers found essentially no differences between the dosed and non-dosed conditions.[275]

Residual Levels of THC

Residual levels of THC are something clinicians who recommend cannabis medicine need to be aware of since one or more of their patients may be charged with driving under the influence (DUI) of cannabis. This may occur even though the police report provides documentation to the contrary. This false charge can be related to elevated blood THC levels resulting from the fat solubility of cannabinoids and the fact that many law enforcement officers are ill-informed regarding cannabis, cannabinoids, and the endocannabinoid system.

Many studies document the phenomenon of THC accumulating in the body's adipose tissue and then being released slowly back into the bloodstream. Agurell et al. studied THC levels in one "heavy marijuana user." His plasma THC was measured each day for four days before and one hour after smoking one cigarette laced with 10 mg radioactively labeled THC and for eight days after ceasing all cannabis use. Prior to the experiment, his plasma THC was roughly 20 mg/ml. The levels of labeled and unlabeled THC both rose after smoking each cigarette, indicating the existing THC may be displaced from the fatty tissues as fresh THC is absorbed.[276]

---

[274] Robbe, H. W. J. "Marijuana's effects on actual driving performance." Adelaide, Australia: Kloeden C, McLean AJ, editors (1995).

[275] Lamers, Caroline TJ, and Johannes Gerardus Ramaekers. "Visual search and urban driving under the influence of marijuana and alcohol." *Human Psychopharmacology: Clinical and Experimental* 16, no. 5 (2001): 393-401.

[276] Lindgren, Jan-Erik, Agneta Ohlsson, Stig Agurell, Leo Hollister, and Hamp Gillespie. "Clinical effects and plasma levels of Δ-9-tetrahydrocannabinol (Δ-9-THC) in heavy and light users of cannabis."

Part III: Cannabis for Clinicians

This part of the book addresses the body of evidence that supports the involvement of the endocannabinoid system in the pathophysiology of several diseases, as well as studies that point to the therapeutic potential of cannabis.

Introduction to the Medical Use of Cannabis

The use of phytocannabinoids for medicinal purposes has been recognized by humankind for millennia. Research has dissected and deepened the scientific understanding of these therapeutic effects for at least 50 years. The results have corroborated the understanding of the therapeutic potential and limitations of phytocannabinoids as a medicine.

The ECS is a critical system within the human body. It is responsible for numerous physiological, metabolic, psychological, and pathological functions. However, it has only been identified and described in the last 30 years, and very few medical schools even mention its existence. Unfortunately, the politicization of the cannabis plant has prevented the clinical trials necessary to provide medical professionals with evidence-based guidelines to guide clinical incorporation.

Over the past 20 years, research seeking to understand the ECS and its interaction with plant components and other synthetic molecules has increased quickly. However, as with the use of opioids, the lack of research does not seem to prevent consumption, and thus, phytocannabinoids have been widely used around the planet for a range of therapeutic purposes—with or without professional medical guidance.

Several barriers are preventing medical professionals from incorporating cannabis into medical practice. Dose adjustment and minimizing potential adverse effects are the two most significant. Some patients report satisfactory effects with a small amount of phytocannabinoids, while others use quite high doses to obtain the same effects. Dosage is incredibly variable: some patients may attain a therapeutic dose of as little as one milligram per day, while others may require as much as two grams per day without the presence of adverse events. The dose-response curve, in general, shows a common bell-shaped pattern in which the desired effect is obtained at medium doses, while at the extremes of the curve, the same effect is not observed.[277,278]

---

[277] Russo, E. B. (2011). "Taming THC: potential cannabis synergy and phytocannabinoid-terpenoid entourage effects." *British Journal of Pharmacology, 163*(7), 1344–1364. https://doi.org/10.1111/j.1476-5381.2011.01238.x

[278] Russo, E. B., & Marcu, J. P. (2017a). "Cannabis Pharmacology: the usual suspects and a few promising leads." In *Advances in pharmacology* (pp. 67–134). https://doi.org/10.1016/bs.apha.2017.03.004

Oral ingestion of doses greater than 10 mg of THC can promote anxiety, dysphoria, psychotic symptoms, physical and mental sedation, euphoria, and tachycardia. The physiological, mental, and subjective effects of experiencing high THC levels are conditioned by the presence of other phytocannabinoids, such as CBD. This interaction may exacerbate some of the effects of THC and may also mitigate other effects, such as anxiety, psychotic symptoms, and cognitive impairment. The same variety of cannabis with the same profile of phytocannabinoids can trigger opposite effects in different people. Anxiety, for example, can be stimulated or attenuated by exposure to the same concentrations of phytocannabinoids depending on the individual, the context of their use, and the presence of other molecules, such as terpenes. While consumption of one variety may induce sleep, another may prevent it due to these variations.

A highly important phenomenon in plant therapy in general, including cannabis, is the so-called entourage effect, resulting from the interaction of all the phytocompounds present in the plant that act together to create their effects, as opposed to a single-molecule pharmaceutical product. The use of these molecules in association results in an effect that appears to be more lasting, effective, safe, and tolerable than treatment with some of these active principles alone.[279,280,281,282] The chemical composition of cannabis varieties is incredibly diverse and continues to diversify as modern cannabis markets mature. These different cannabis varieties can be categorized by their phytochemical content, referred to as "chemotypes." The dosage, the chemotype, and the method of ingestion (route of administration) play a significant role in the varying effects different people experience, and this part of the book will break this down in further detail.

---

[279] Russo, E. B. (2011). "Taming THC: potential cannabis synergy and phytocannabinoid-terpenoid entourage effects." *British Journal of Pharmacology, 163*(7), 1344–1364. https://doi.org/10.1111/j.1476-5381.2011.01238.x

[280] Ben-Shabat, S., Fride, E., Sheskin, T., Tamiri, T., Rhee, M. H., Vogel, Z., Bisogno, T., De Petrocellis, L., Di Marzo, V., & Mechoulam, R. (1998b). "An entourage effect: inactive endogenous fatty acid glycerol esters enhance 2-arachidonoyl-glycerol cannabinoid activity." *European Journal of Pharmacology, 353*(1), 23–31. https://doi.org/10.1016/s0014-2999(98)00392-6

[281] Pamplona, F. A., Da Silva, L. R., & Coan, A. C. (2018). "Potential Clinical Benefits of CBD-Rich cannabis extracts over Purified CBD in Treatment-Resistant Epilepsy: Observational Data Meta-analysis." *Frontiers in Neurology*, 9. https://doi.org/10.3389/fneur.2018.00759

[282] Bonn-Miller, M. O., ElSohly, M. A., Loflin, M., Chandra, S., & Vandrey, R. G. (2018). "Cannabis and cannabinoid drug development: evaluating botanical versus single molecule approaches." *International Review of Psychiatry, 30*(3), 277–284. https://doi.org/10.1080/09540261.2018.1474730

Although the research to guide clinical incorporation is still lacking, there is significant evidence for the use of cannabis and cannabinoids in the treatment of many pathologies, symptoms, and conditions such as spasticity, cancers in general, nausea and vomiting, rheumatoid arthritis, depression, irritable bowel syndrome, epilepsies in general, symptoms associated with amyotrophic lateral sclerosis (ALS), motor dysfunction and cognitive impairment associated with Huntington's disease, Parkinson's symptoms such as dyskinesia, reduced consumption of other addictive substances, sleep problems, post-traumatic stress disorder, schizophrenia and psychosis, anxiety relief, diabetes and metabolic, immunological, cardiovascular diseases, among others.

Because the lack of evidence does not preclude the empirical use of cannabis and phytocannabinoids, a growing body of case reports and anecdotal testimonials has largely guided its use. This section of the book provides the available research required for doctors to guide their patients or patients to guide themselves, using what is known today while also acknowledging the limitations due to a lack of clinical trials.

Therapeutic Applications of Cannabis

The following list provides a general overview of the known therapeutic applications of cannabis and phytocannabinoids:

- ADHD/attention deficit treatment
- Anti-bacterial
- Anti-nausea/Anti-emetic
- Analgesic
- Anticonvulsant
- Anti-inflammatory
- Anxiolytic
- Antidepressant
- Antispasmodic
- Appetite stimulator
- Bronchodilator
- Apoptosis stimulator
- Inhibits angiogenesis
- Inhibits cancer growth
- Inhibits the Id-1 gene

- Treatment for post-traumatic stress disorder (PTSD)
- Reduces blood glucose levels
- Sleep disorders
- Stimulation of bone growth
- Vasodilation

Conditions in which cannabis can be an adjuvant:

Analgesia
- Intractable pain
- Neuropathic pain
- Osteoarthritis
- Other forms of chronic pain
- Phantom limb pain

Autoimmune Diseases
- Crohn's disease
- Complex regional pain syndrome
- Fibromyalgia
- Systemic lupus erythematosus
- Reflex sympathetic dystrophy
- Rheumatoid arthritis
- Scleroderma

Endocannabinoid Deficiency Syndrome
- Attention deficit disorder
- Attention deficit hyperactivity disorder (ADHD)
- Autistic Spectrum Disorder (ASD)
- Asperger's syndrome
- Social anxiety
- Obsessive-compulsive disorder (OCD)
- Bipolar disorder
- Crohn's disease
- Explosive disorder
- Panic syndrome
- Tourette's Syndrome

Gastrointestinal
- Anorexia
- Appetite stimulation
- Inflammatory bowel disease, ulcerative colitis and Crohn's disease
- Nausea

Mental Health
- Attention deficit disorder
- Anger management issues
- Anxiety
- Bipolar disorder
- Depression
- Hypervigilance syndrome
- Impulse control issues
- Mood disorders
- OCD
- Panic attacks
- PTSD
- Stress relief

Motor Control
- Dystonia
- Essential tremor
- Multiple sclerosis (MS)
- Parkinson's disease (PD)
- Tourette's syndrome

Neurodegenerative Disease / Neurodegeneration
(see also: Motor Control)
- Alzheimer's disease (AD)
- Amyotrophic lateral sclerosis (ALS) (Lou Gehrig's Disease)
- Cerebellar degeneration
- Huntington's disease (HD)
- Multiple sclerosis
- Parkinson's disease

Others/General
- AIDS—pain/appetite
- Addiction/substitute for harm reduction
- Asthma
- Cancer
- Epilepsy and seizures
- Insomnia and other sleep disorders
- Migraine
- Sickness
- Neuroprotective effect
- PTSD
- Pain relief
- Skin conditions
- Spinal cord injury
- Stroke and traumatic brain injury (TBI).

Summary of the Medicinal Effects of Cannabis Resin[283]

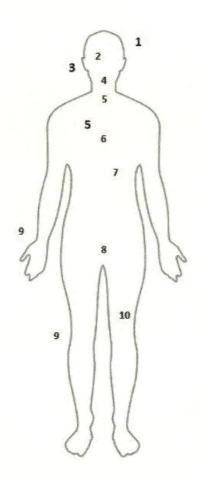

1. The brain absorbs THC through unique sites on the receptor that affects body systems, activating a chain of temporary physiological and psychological effects. It initially has a stimulating effect, followed by relaxation and general stress reduction. May cause drowsiness or anxiety. Analgesic effect (decreased pain). Blocks migraines or seizures. Increases sense of well-being.
2. Cannabis reddens and dehydrates the eyes.
3. Ringing in the ears (tinnitus).
4. Dehydrates the mouth and stimulates the appetite.
5. Has an expectorant effect, clearing the throat and lungs.
6. Accelerates heart rate and pulse rate. Dilates bronchi and blood vessels.
7. Calms the stomach. Stimulates the appetite. Restores the gastrointestinal tract. Reduces nausea (antiemetic) and vomiting. Helps with motion sickness and alleviates various adverse effects of radiation and chemotherapy.
8. Little or no effect on the reproductive system. No proven mutagenic effects. Traditionally used as an aphrodisiac and for impotence.
9. Soothes the joints. General analgesic effect and pain reducer. Anti-inflammatory that helps with arthritis and rheumatism when given orally or by topical application. Vasodilation carries blood faster from the extremities, lowering the overall body temperature.

---

[283] *Hemp for Health: The Medicinal and Nutritional Uses of Cannabis Sativa: Conrad, Chris: 9780892815395: Amazon.com: Books.* (n.d.). https://www.amazon.com/Hemp-Health-Medicinal-Nutritional-Cannabis/dp/0892815396

10. Relaxes muscles. Reduces muscle cramps, seizures, spasms, ataxia, and other neurological or movement disorders.
11. Helps mitigate or control symptoms of multiple sclerosis (MS), spinal injury, and epilepsy.
12. Body fat tissue collects inert cannabinoids for removal.

The following chapters in this section provide more insight on how doctors, clinicians, and other healthcare professionals can incorporate cannabis into clinical practice as well as a summary of current research for conditions patients most frequently turn to cannabis or cannabinoid-based medicines to treat.

Integrative Medicine

With progressive frequency, health professionals have been sought by patients with chronic conditions that, moreover, do not respond to conventional treatments. In this context, the effectiveness of **allopathic** medicines has its applicability questioned, and, therefore, new ways of practicing and understanding care become necessary. The **integrative** approach has been identified as a more effective way of treating patients, especially those with chronic illnesses.[284]

Integrative care is a comprehensive treatment model that considers the human body as an indivisible entity. Thus, the approach is to integrate different clinical specialties and adapt them according to the individuality and needs of each patient, not focusing exclusively on the presented complaint but on the conditions that led to it being expressed.[285]

By analyzing health and the factors that can harm it, this approach allows one to aim at preventing certain conditions and their necessary care. In this way, it also proves to be a more accessible, cost-effective care tool for the patient.[286]

In addition to considering the physical aspects of complaints, illnesses, and conditions, the integrative approach also focuses on the patient's emotional, psychological, and social aspects, emphasizing disease prevention and health promotion. Its space in clinics has been growing, especially as an investigation technique for chronic diseases. To this end, complementary therapies paired with conventional medicine are combined to remedy the complaints presented or even improve the patient's quality of life, mitigating their complaints or reducing symptoms of anxiety, depression, and need for medication.[287]

Despite including therapies with passively-acquired benefits (through practices such as acupuncture and massage), the practice also calls for lifestyle changes and the inclusion of active therapeutic habits such as meditation, yoga, and nutritional changes. These practices, as stated, aim to

---

[284] Jonas, W. B., & Rosenbaum, E. (2021). "The case for Whole-Person Integrative care." *Medicina-lithuania*, 57(7), 677. https://doi.org/10.3390/medicina57070677

[285] Fan, D. (2017). "Holistic integrative medicine: toward a new era of medical advancement." *Frontiers of Medicine*, 11(1), 152–159. https://doi.org/10.1007/s11684-017-0499-6

[286] Guarneri, E., Horrigan, B., & Pechura, C. M. (2010). "The Efficacy and Cost Effectiveness of Integrative Medicine: A review of the medical and Corporate literature." *Explore-the Journal of Science and Healing*, 6(5), 308–312. https://doi.org/10.1016/j.explore.2010.06.012

[287] SBMI – Sociedade Brasileira de Medicina Integrativa. (n.d.). http://sbmi.org.br/

complement conventional practice, bringing additional benefits to the patient.[288]

According to the Brazilian Society of Integrative Medicine:

[Integrative medicine] is a medical practice that uses different therapies to promote health, prevent diseases, treat organic and emotional imbalances, and integrate scientific and cultural knowledge from different medical areas.

It is important to emphasize that in addition to bringing benefits in an active, passive, and complementary way, the practice also seeks to engage patients by allowing them to assume the leadership role in their health care. This engagement helps to break the paradigm of "the physician as the protagonist and possessor of the panacea capable of curing all health conditions."

Changes in behavior and food habits are a significant part of the patient's appropriation and autonomy over their health. In this way, it is possible to implement changes and adaptations in habits with gradual introductions and alterations because, precisely concerning integrative care, it is extremely important that patients and caregivers take the reins of planning, development, and application of strategies they shape with healthcare professionals.

Immunity is negatively impacted by Western lifestyle and diet. Although low, the level of endogenous inflammation resulting from food is persistent, and due to its relationship with intestinal health and the functioning of the microbiota, it is vital to use a diet rich in vegetable fibers, antioxidants, and healthy fats. Integrative practice associates the adoption of these habits with the use of specific bacterial strains (contained in probiotics) to positively alter the absorption of nutrients from the patient's new health habits.[289]

For success with integrative medicine, patients must be willing to actively participate in their own care. Consider the words of Hippocrates:

Before healing someone, ask them if they are willing to give up the things that made them sick.

For the personalized care application, adaptation of behaviors, potential optimization of the health situation, and improvement of quality of life, the

---

[288] "BRASIL Ministério da Saúde. Política Nacional de Práticas Integrativas e Complementares no SUS." Brasília: Ministério da Saúde, 2006. Disponível em: http://bvsms.saude.gov.br/bvs/publicacoes/politica_nacional_praticas_integrativas_complementares.pdf

[289] Bengmark, S. (2012). "Integrative medicine and human health - the role of pre-, pro- and synbiotics." *Clinical and Translational Medicine*, 1(1). https://doi.org/10.1186/2001-1326-1-6

patient-protagonist must be willing to consider changes in their habits in favor of aiding their complaints. In addition to seeking to mitigate the complaints presented, the integrative approach also aims to prevent other potential conditions that may be harmful in the long term.

By raising the previous question about Hippocrates's reflection, it is possible to start an investigation of the factors that can lead to illness or worsening of pre-existing health conditions through three specific layers in the patient's life experience:[290]

- **Thought:** Employ practices that strengthen awareness and self-knowledge, including understanding and respecting one's limits, wills, and capabilities. Integrative medicine envisions employing practices such as meditation[291] to improve a patient's quality of life, focus, and overall well-being. In addition to encouraging contact with oneself and concentrating on the present moment, this practice promotes self-knowledge, an essential tool for understanding, welcoming, and direction. And this is not limited to health alone. Working on "thought" also means practicing sleep hygiene and reducing factors that contribute to anxiety. Furthermore, it empowers the patient to take responsibility for improving their health condition.
- **Food:** The reduction and/or exclusion of foods that are potentially harmful to health, as well as the use of nutritional supplementation and probiotic complementation when necessary, is a pillar of the integrative approach.[292] Excessive consumption of milk and gluten, as well as their derivatives, can trigger discomfort even in patients who do not have an intolerance or celiac disease, and to mitigate these conditions, it is recommended to reduce food and products derived from these components[293] as they also have the potential to aggravate pre-existing conditions. Avoid processed foods, especially refined oils, sugars, and grains.

---

[290] Schestatsky P. "Medicina do amanhã: como a genética, o estilo de vida e a tecnologia juntos podem auxiliar na sua qualidade de vida." São Paulo: Gente, 2021.

[291] Esch, T. (2021). "Meditation in Complementary and Integrative Medicine: Taxonomy of Effects and Methods." *Complementary Medicine Research*, 28(3), 183–187. https://doi.org/10.1159/000516849

[292] Bolte, L. A., Vila, A. V., Imhann, F., Collij, V., Gaćeša, R., Peters, V., Wijmenga, C., Kurilshikov, A., Campmans-Kuijpers, M. J. E., Fu, J., Dijkstra, G., Zhernakova, A., & Weersma, R. K. (2021). "Long-term dietary patterns are associated with pro-inflammatory and anti-inflammatory features of the gut microbiome." *Gut*, 70(7), 1287–1298. https://doi.org/10.1136/gutjnl-2020-322670

[293] Bernstein, C. D., Gillman, A. G., Zhang, D., Bartman, A. E., Jeong, J., & Wasan, A. D. (2020). "Identifying predictors of recommendations for and participation in multimodal nonpharmacological treatments for chronic pain using Patient-Reported Outcomes and Electronic medical records." *Pain Medicine*. https://doi.org/10.1093/pm/pnaa203

- **Movement:** It is essential to underline the importance of the practice of physical exercises. Physical health can also be optimized through practices such as acupuncture and massage.

Analgesia

The number one symptom of most diseases, conditions, and illnesses is pain. Many patients who obtain a doctor's recommendation for cannabis or even visit an adult use (legal) dispensary seek cannabis for its pain-relieving effects, whether from temporary symptomatic pain or chronic pain due to injury or illness. There is consistent evidence for chronic pain relief with cannabinoid therapy.[294] Considering the toll of the opiate epidemic, much attention has been paid to cannabis as an alternative.

Several constituents of cannabis contribute to its analgesic effects. These constituents include THC, CBD, CBN, CBG, CBC, and several terpenes, including myrcene, limonene, borneol, β-caryophyllene, α-pinene, and linalool. Cannabinoids can decrease the frequency of pain signals through retrograde inhibition. By slowing the speed of neurotransmission, the brain receives fewer pain signals. An increase in cannabinoids also causes the cannabinoid-modulated central pain interpretation center (one of two such pain centers—the other is mediated by the endorphins) to interpret pain as less severe. Many patients say that they have less pain, and some say they still have the pain, but it is easier to concentrate on something else, yet still others say that it is a combination of the two.

> A team of researchers at the University of Washington developed educational models regarding the use of cannabis for chronic pain. Healthcare professionals can utilize these modules and earn continuing education credits for a nominal fee. These modules can be viewed for free on their website.[295]

Cannabis-Like Substances in the Brain Relieve Pain

As long ago as 1999, a report on the proceedings of the National Academy of Sciences, Marijuana as Medicine: Assessing the Science Base, stated, "US researchers report that pain triggers the release of a marijuana-like chemical called anandamide deep in the brain that works as a natural pain reliever. Anandamide levels in the brain also rose significantly in response to painful

---

[294] Campos, R. M. P., Aguiar, A. F. L., Paes-Colli, Y., Trindade, P. M. P., Ferreira, B. K., De Melo Reis, R. A., & Sampaio, L. S. (2021). "Cannabinoid therapeutics in chronic neuropathic pain: From animal research to human treatment." *Frontiers in Physiology, 12.* https://doi.org/10.3389/fphys.2021.785176

[295] https://adai.uw.edu/mcacp/index.htm

stimuli."[296] "The fall in pain perception was paralleled by a significant rise in the levels of anandamide in a portion of the brain called the periaqueductal gray, or PAG. The increase of anandamide in the PAG resulted in greatly diminished pain sensitivity in rats. The rats' pain perception returned to normal after being administered a substance that blocked anandamide."[297] This study supports a second endocannabinoid-mediated pain interpretation center in the brain, other than that mediated by endorphins. The report also hypothesizes that these results, when taken together, support the existence of a pain control system within the periaqueductal gray region (PAG).

The report goes on to state that this pain control center "...is triggered by pain and promotes analgesia through the release of anandamide." Consistent with these findings, the researchers suggest that drugs that affect the endocannabinoid system might form the basis of a modern approach to the treatment of pain.

Consistent with these findings, the researchers suggest that drugs that affect the ECS could form the basis of a modern approach to pain management. In fact, a study of 300 patients by the American Academy of Cannabinoid Medicine (AACM) revealed that pain relief is the number one reason for cannabinoid use by medical experts who recommend the use of cannabis. In addition, systematized questionnaires and user self-reports indicate that chronic pain is the main interest in cannabinoid therapy. In US states that have regulated access to cannabinoids, there has been a considerable decrease in the prescription of other pain medications,[298] including a significant reduction in deaths from opioids compared to other states where therapeutic cannabis is not available and regulated.[299] However, many

---

[296] Joy, Janet, Stanley J. Watson, Jr., and John A. Benson, eds. *Marijuana and Medicine: Assessing the Science Base Washington D.C.*: National Academy Press, 1999

[297] Walker, J. Michael, Susan M. Huang, Nicole M. Strangman, Kang Tsou, and M. Clara Sañudo-Peña. "Pain modulation by release of the endogenous cannabinoid anandamide." Proceedings of the National Academy of Sciences 96, no. 21 (1999): 12198-12203

[298] National Academies of Sciences, Engineering, and Medicine, 2017.

[299] Bachhuber, M. A., Saloner, B., Cunningham, C. O., & Barry, C. L. (2014). "Medical Cannabis Laws and opioid analgesic overdose mortality in the United States, 1999-2010." *JAMA Internal Medicine, 174*(10), 1668. https://doi.org/10.1001/jamainternmed.2014.4005

studies warn that adverse events caused by THC may still negatively influence treatment.[300,301]

A clinical, multicenter, parallel, double-blind, randomized, and placebo-controlled trial evaluated the effectiveness of associating THC with CBD for cancer pain. The same trial demonstrated that the treatment was able to significantly reduce pain scores by more than 30% compared to placebo.[302] Other clinical studies have demonstrated treatment efficacy in reducing neuropathic pain symptoms through the consumption of inhaled phytocannabinoids.[303,304] Meta-analysis studies point to the effectiveness of treating neuropathic pain in patients with MS. The data also show the significant effect of treatment with phytocannabinoids, either by absorption of the extract through the oral mucosa or by inhaled use, compared to placebo.[305,306]

A Cochrane review evaluated the efficacy and safety of clinical trials for neuropathic pain with cannabis-derived drugs. This study pointed out a 30% reduction in pain symptoms. The study considered the grade of evidence to

---

[300] Koppel, B. S., Brust, J. C., Fife, T. D., Bronstein, J. M., Youssof, S., Gronseth, G. S., & Gloss, D. (2014). "Systematic review: Efficacy and safety of medical marijuana in selected neurologic disorders: Report of the Guideline Development Subcommittee of the American Academy of Neurology." *Neurology*, 82(17), 1556–1563. https://doi.org/10.1212/wnl.0000000000000363

[301] Mücke, M., Phillips, T. E., Radbruch, L., Petzke, F., & Häuser, W. (2018). "Cannabis-based medicines for chronic neuropathic pain in adults." The Cochrane Library, 2020(7). https://doi.org/10.1002/14651858.cd012182.pub2

[302] Johnson, J. J., Burnell-Nugent, M., Lossignol, D., Ganae-Motan, E. D. E., Potts, R. R., & Fallon, M. (2010). "Multicenter, Double-Blind, Randomized, Placebo-Controlled, Parallel-Group Study of the Efficacy, Safety, and Tolerability of THC:CBD Extract and THC Extract in Patients with Intractable Cancer-Related Pain." *Journal of Pain and Symptom Management*, 39(2), 167–179. https://doi.org/10.1016/j.jpainsymman.2009.06.008

[303] Abrams, D. I., Jay, C. A., Shade, S. B., Vizoso, H., Reda, H., Press, S., Kelly, M. E., Rowbotham, M. C., & Petersen, K. L. (2007). "Cannabis in painful HIV-associated sensory neuropathy: A randomized placebo-controlled trial." *Neurology*, 68(7), 515–521. https://doi.org/10.1212/01.wnl.0000253187.66183.9c

[304] Ware, M. A., Wang, T., Shapiro, S., Ducruet, T., Huynh, T., Gamsa, A., Bennett, G. J., & Collet, J. (2010). "Smoked cannabis for chronic neuropathic pain: a randomized controlled trial." *Canadian Medical Association Journal*, 182(14), E694–E701. https://doi.org/10.1503/cmaj.091414

[305] Iskedjian M, Bereza B, Gordon A, Piwko C, Einarson TR. "Meta-analysis of cannabis based treatments for neuropathic and multiple sclerosis-related pain." Curr Med Res Opin. 2007 Jan;23(1):17-24. doi: 10.1185/030079906x158066. PMID: 17257464.

[306] Andreae, M. H., Carter, G. M., Shaparin, N., Sandberg, K., Ellis, R. J., Ware, M. A., Abrams, D. I., Prasad, H., Wilsey, B., Indyk, D., Johnson, M. S., & Sacks, H. S. (2015). "Inhaled cannabis for Chronic Neuropathic pain: A Meta-analysis of individual patient data." *The Journal of Pain*, 16(12), 1221–1232. https://doi.org/10.1016/j.jpain.2015.07.009

be of moderate quality for this treatment.[307] Another meta-analysis study[308] that evaluated 79 clinical trials related to the use of cannabinoids for therapeutic purposes found a moderate degree of quality of evidence regarding cannabinoids' efficacy. Patients showed about 40% improvement in pain when compared to the placebo group.[309] Other researchers criticize the lack of data and experiments that can more consistently elucidate the use of cannabinoids for pain treatment. These also point out that new regulatory scenarios should encourage risk-benefit assessment research of this treatment so that there is proof of its viability.[310]

More Research on the Analgesic Properties of Cannabis

There is a wealth of research about the pain-relieving effects of cannabis and this chapter does not attempt to summarize them all. However, it does take a close look at some of the most influential studies that can guide the clinical use of cannabis as an analgesic medicine.

Institute of Medicine

There is a substantial body of anecdotal and research-based evidence of the analgesic properties of cannabis. In 1982 the Institute of Medicine (IOM) reported, "Several animal models have been used to show analgesic effects of cannabis and its analogues." As examples, they cited Grunfeld and Edery, 1969, Sofia et al, 1973, and Noyes et al., 1976. Each of these studies found a reduction in pain reports by cancer patients given oral Δ^9-THC.[311]

The 1999 IOM report on medical cannabis "Marijuana and Medicine: Assessing the Science Base" stated, "The accumulated data indicate a

---

[307] Mücke, M., Phillips, T. E., Radbruch, L., Petzke, F., & Häuser, W. (2018). "Cannabis-based medicines for chronic neuropathic pain in adults." *The Cochrane Library*, 2020(7). https://doi.org/10.1002/14651858.cd012182.pub2

[308] Nielsen, S., Germanos, R., Weier, M., Pollard, J. D., Degenhardt, L., Hall, W., Buckley, N. A., & Farrell, M. (2018). "The Use of Cannabis and Cannabinoids in Treating Symptoms of Multiple Sclerosis: a Systematic Review of Reviews." *Current Neurology and Neuroscience Reports*, 18(2). https://doi.org/10.1007/s11910-018-0814-x

[309] Joy, J. E., Watson, S. J., & Benson, J. (1999). "Marijuana and medicine." In *National Academies Press eBooks*. https://doi.org/10.17226/6376

[310] Hill, K. P., Palastro, M. D., Johnson, B., & Ditre, J. W. (2017). "Cannabis and Pain: A clinical review." *Cannabis and Cannabinoid Research*, 2(1), 96–104. https://doi.org/10.1089/can.2017.0017

[311] "GW Pharmaceuticals Achieves Positive Results in Phase 2 Proof of Concept Study in Glioma," GW Pharmaceuticals. https://www.gwpharm.com/about-us/news/gw-pharmaceuticals-achieves-positive-results-phase-2-proof-concept-study-glioma

potential therapeutic value for cannabinoid drugs, particularly for symptoms such as pain relief, control of nausea and vomiting, and appetite stimulation."[312] They concluded that cannabis had medical value and that its side effects were similar to the bulk of prescription drugs then on the market.

Society for Neuroscience

In 1997, a *Los Angeles Times* article reported on several studies presented at the Society for Neuroscience addressing the painkilling properties of cannabis. These studies were done at such institutions as the University of Texas, the University of Minnesota, Brown University, Wake Forest School of Medicine, and the University of California at San Francisco (UCSF). According to the *Times* article, researchers reported that "active chemicals found in the plant could serve as an effective remedy for the millions who suffer serious pain each year without the unwanted side effects of more traditional morphine-like drugs."[313]

California Center for Medicinal Cannabis Research (CMCR)

Since 2001, the center located at the University of California at San Diego (UCSD) School of Medicine has coordinated and supported cannabis research throughout the state. Initially, four diseases or conditions were designated as areas of emphasis for CMCR funding. One symptom was chronic pain, particularly neuropathic pain. In 2011 the CMCR released a summary of the 18 FDA-approved clinically related studies completed at four UC medical schools. At least five of these studies were related to pain relief, and at least two were published in peer-reviewed medical journals. Since 2015, cannabis research centers have been instituted at the University of California Los Angeles and the University of California Irvine Schools of Medicine.

University of New Mexico

University of New Mexico researchers evaluated prescription drug use patterns over a 24-month period. They compared opiate use in 83 pain patients enrolled in the state's medical cannabis program to 42 non-enrolled patients. The study reported that 36% of the program registrants significantly reduced their prescription drug intake while non-registrants diagnosed with similar conditions did not. Furthermore, by the study's end, 34% of registered

---

[312] Joy, Janet, Stanley J. Watson, Jr., and John A. Benson, eds. *Marijuana and Medicine: Assessing the Science Base.* Washington D.C.: National Academy Press, 1999.

[313] "Chemicals in Pot Cut Severe Pain, Study Says." *Los Angeles Times.* Last Modified October 27, 1997.

cannabis program patients had eliminated their use of prescription drugs altogether.³¹⁴

NORML wrote, "Legal access to cannabis may reduce the use of multiple classes of dangerous prescription medications in certain patient populations." They concluded, "[a] shift from prescriptions for other scheduled drugs to cannabis may result in less frequent interactions with our conventional healthcare system and potentially improved patient health."³¹⁵

Cost Savings

A study published in the journal *Health Affairs* reported that medical cannabis access is associated with lower Medicaid expenditures and Medicare Part D-approved prescription medications.³¹⁶ In 2017 *Forbes* reported on the findings by Ashley C. Bradford and W. David Bradford, who analyzed data from 2007-2014 that concluded that if "all states had legalized medical marijuana in 2014, Medicaid could have saved $1 billion in spending on prescriptions."³¹⁷

National Institute on Drug Abuse (NIDA)

Nora Volkow, MD, director of NIDA and a longtime skeptic of cannabis's medicinal properties, was the keynote speaker at the 2017 American Society of Addiction Medicine (ASAM) meeting. Dr. Volkow spoke on strategies for dealing with the opiate epidemic. Her first bullet point was to tell the addictionologists present at the conference that, when possible, cannabis should be recommended for pain relief rather than prescribing an opiate.

---

³¹⁴ Stith, Sarah S., Jacob M. Vigil, Ian Marshall Adams, and Anthony P. Reeve. "Effects of Legal Access to Cannabis on Scheduled II-V Drug Prescriptions." Journal of the American Medical Directors Association 19, no. 1 (2018): 59-64

³¹⁵ "Study: Medical Marijuana Legalization Linked to Lower Medicaid Costs." NORML. April 27, 2017. http://norml.org/news/2017/04/27/study-medical-marijuana-legalization-linked-to-lower-medicaid-costs/

³¹⁶ *Ibid*

³¹⁷ Borchardt, D. (2017, April 21). Medicaid could have saved $1 billion if medical marijuana was legalized. Forbes. https://www.forbes.com/sites/debraborchardt/2017/04/21/medicaid-could-have-saved-1-billion-if-medical-marijuana-was-legalized/?sh=2a894fb47c57

Autoimmune Diseases

Autoimmune diseases are chronic conditions characterized by the immune system attacking healthy cells, tissues, and organs. There are more than 80 defined autoimmune diseases, the most common of which are Type 1 diabetes, multiple sclerosis, rheumatoid arthritis, lupus, Crohn's disease, and psoriasis. These conditions are often treated with anti-inflammatory drugs, corticosteroids, or other pharmaceutical treatments that generally treat the symptoms, rather than the underlying cause, of the disease. For this reason, many of the first and most vocal patients in state-legal medical cannabis programs were and continue to be autoimmune patients. Many use cannabis for the relief of pain, insomnia, anxiety, or nausea associated with their diagnosis. In some cases, they profess the curative or treatment properties of cannabis for some of the more serious symptoms of their disease, such as the spasticity associated with multiple sclerosis or digestive upset associated with Crohn's disease. This chapter takes a closer look at the **pathophysiology** of three such diseases—Crohn's disease, psoriasis, and multiple sclerosis—as well as the therapeutic potential of cannabis and cannabinoids in their treatment.

Crohn's Disease

Crohn's disease (CD) is a chronic inflammatory disease of the gastrointestinal tract that can result in fistulas, which are abnormal connections between organs, or strictures, which are blockages in the intestines that require surgical resection. The most common symptoms are diarrhea, abdominal pain, weight loss, presence of blood or mucus in the sputum, and perianal pain, which may be associated with the occurrence of arthritis, uveitis, and skin rashes.[318,319]

The mechanism involved in CD's pathophysiological process involves a gene studied by Hammer et al.[320] known as the HLA-B27/β2 microglobulin. According to the bacterial hypothesis, chronic inflammation may be related

---

[318] Carter, M. J., Lobo, A., & Travis, S. (2004). "Guidelines for the management of inflammatory bowel disease in adults." *Gut, 53*(suppl_5), v1–v16. https://doi.org/10.1136/gut.2004.043372

[319] Travis, S. (2006). "European evidence based consensus on the diagnosis and management of Crohn's disease: current management." *Gut, 55*(suppl_1), i16–i35. https://doi.org/10.1136/gut.2005.081950b

[320] Hammer, R. E., Maika, S. D., Richardson, J. A., Tang, J. P., & Taurog, J. D. (1990). Spontaneous inflammatory disease in transgenic rats expressing HLA-B27 and human β2m: An animal model of HLA-B27-associated human disorders. *Cell, 63*(5), 1099–1112. https://doi.org/10.1016/0092-8674(90)90512-d

to the microbiota, where the intestinal membrane and the synovial membrane express the same receptors.[321]

The process of chronic inflammation in CD, as well as in other pathologies, is related to increased levels of **reactive oxygen species (ROS)**, which are unpaired molecules responsible for favoring the development of chronic diseases through the disordered balance between their formation and antioxidants present in the body or from food. With the intracellular increase of ROS, NF-κB phosphorylation and activation of the COX2 inflammation pathway is triggered, leading to the activation of PGH2 and PGE2 prostaglandins and, consequently, to the release of pro-inflammatory cytokines, such as IL-6, as shown in the figure below. Antioxidant defense mechanisms involve the activity of superoxide dismutase (SOD) and catalase (CAT) enzymes present in the intracellular environment. SOD neutralizes ROS into hydrogen peroxide, which is then transformed into water and oxygen by CAT. The exacerbated production of cytokines leads to the recruitment of cells of the inflammatory system, whose metabolism produces ROS, generating more inflammation, leading to a repetitive cycle.[322,323]

The clinical diagnosis of CD consists of evaluating symptoms such as abdominal pain, fever, and long-lasting diarrhea with periods of activity and remission.[324] There are also some risk factors, such as genetic predisposition, high consumption of total fats, fatty acids, omega-6, and red meat, as well as smoking, aggravating the clinical condition of the patient. CD significantly affects patient quality of life, with at least 50% of patients with CD undergoing surgical intervention during the first ten years of the disease, in addition to developing a predisposition to colorectal cancer.[325]

Pharmacological treatment of CD involves the use of non-steroidal anti-inflammatory drugs (NSAIDs), which can inhibit the COX enzyme and,

---

[321] Taurog, J. D., Richardson, J. A., Croft, J., Simmons, W. A., Zhou, M., Fernández-Sueiro, J. L., Balish, E., & Hammer, R. E. (1994). "The germfree state prevents development of gut and joint inflammatory disease in HLA-B27 transgenic rats." *Journal of Experimental Medicine*, 180(6), 2359–2364. https://doi.org/10.1084/jem.180.6.2359

[322] Mittal, M., Siddiqui, M. R., Tran, K. A., Reddy, S. P., & Malik, A. B. (2014). "Reactive oxygen species in inflammation and tissue injury." *Antioxidants & Redox Signaling*, 20(7), 1126–1167. https://doi.org/10.1089/ars.2012.5149

[323] Blaser, H., Dostert, C., Mak, T. W., & Brenner, D. (2016). "TNF and ROS Crosstalk in Inflammation." *Trends in Cell Biology*, 26(4), 249–261. https://doi.org/10.1016/j.tcb.2015.12.002

[324] Mills, S. C. (2011). *Crohn's disease*. PubMed Central (PMC). https://www.ncbi.nlm.nih.gov/pmc/articles/PMC3217808/

[325] Von Roon, A. C., Reese, G., Teare, J., Constantinides, V., Darzi, A., & Tekkis, P. (2007). "The Risk of Cancer in Patients with Crohn's Disease." *Diseases of the Colon & Rectum*, 50(6), 839–855. https://doi.org/10.1007/s10350-006-0848-z

consequently, NF-κB activity, thus reducing inflammation of the gastrointestinal mucosa.[326] Aminosalicylates, antibiotics, corticosteroids, and immunomodulators are also used.

Phytocannabinoids and Crohn's Disease

Recent studies show that endocannabinoids can inhibit the release of pro-inflammatory mediators, including IL-1, TNF-α, and NO.[327] Activation of CB2 receptors leads to apoptosis of T cells, decreasing their proliferation, and the recruitment of neutrophils and macrophages to the inflamed tissue. Furthermore, CB1 receptors, in turn, participate in intestinal motility control and secretion, decreasing the hypersecretion caused by CD.[328]

A study was conducted with 21 patients with CD who were unresponsive to steroids and immunosuppressant therapy. For eight weeks, the patients received medicinal cannabis flowers containing 115 mg of THC, and the placebo group received cannabis flowers where the compound had been extracted. According to the Crohn's Disease Activity Index (CDAI), the results showed a total remission (CDAI > 150) achieved in five out of 11 patients in the group that used cannabis, in addition to a clinical response (CDAI < 100) in ten out of 11 patients (90%) in the cannabis group compared to the placebo group (four out of 10 patients; 40%). About three patients achieved complete withdrawal from steroid dependence, and all reported increased appetite and sleep without side effects.[329]

Cannabinoids have pharmacological actions on epithelial and immune system cells, resulting in protective and immunomodulatory effects.[330] The THC molecule is considered a partial and non-selective agonist.[331]

---

[326] Cabré, E. (2012). "Impact of environmental and dietary factors on the course of inflammatory bowel disease." *World Journal of Gastroenterology*, 18(29), 3814. https://doi.org/10.3748/wjg.v18.i29.3814

[327] Esposito, G., De Filippis, D., Cirillo, C., Iuvone, T., Capoccia, E., Scuderi, C., Steardo, A., Cuomo, R., & Steardo, L. (2012). "Cannabidiol in Inflammatory bowel Diseases: A brief Overview." *Phytotherapy Research*, 27(5), 633–636. https://doi.org/10.1002/ptr.4781

[328] Schicho, R., & Storr, M. (2013). "Patients with IBD find symptom relief in the Cannabis field." *Nature Reviews Gastroenterology & Hepatology*, 11(3), 142–143. https://doi.org/10.1038/nrgastro.2013.245

[329] Naftali, T., Schleider, L. B., Dotan, I., Lansky, E. P., Benjaminov, F., & Konikoff, F. M. (2013). "Cannabis induces a clinical response in patients with Crohn's Disease: a prospective Placebo-Controlled study." *Clinical Gastroenterology and Hepatology*, 11(10), 1276-1280.e1. https://doi.org/10.1016/j.cgh.2013.04.034

[330] Greineisen, W. E., & Turner, H. (2010). "Immunoactive effects of cannabinoids: Considerations for the therapeutic use of cannabinoid receptor agonists and antagonists." *International Immunopharmacology*, 10(5), 547–555. https://doi.org/10.1016/j.intimp.2010.02.012

[331] Schwilke, E. W., Schwope, D. M., Karschner, E. L., Lowe, R. H., Darwin, W. D., Kelly, D. L., Goodwin, R. S., Gorelick, D. A., & Huestis, M. A. (2009). "Δ9-Tetrahydrocannabinol (THC), 11-Hydroxy-THC, and 11-Nor-9-

Endocannabinoids such as palmitoylethanolamide have pleiotropic effects in the body, including the gastrointestinal tract.[332] AEA, 2-Arachidonoylglycerol ether (noladin ether) and arachidonoylchlorpropamide (ACPA) induce repair systems in colonic epithelial cells, suggesting a curative effect on possible tissue damage caused in CD.[333] Additionally, *in vitro* studies have shown mechanisms in both receptors modulating inflammation, among other mechanisms, such as suppression of macrophage and mast cell activation, secretion of pro-inflammatory cytokines, modulation of helper T lymphocytes by reducing the activation of the T cell population, inducing apoptosis, and inhibiting cell proliferation.[334] In the study by Alhamoruni et al,[335] it was observed that the endocannabinoids AEA and 2-AG increased intestinal permeability when applied to human colon adenocarcinoma cells (Caco-2).

---

carboxy-THC Plasma Pharmacokinetics during and after Continuous High-Dose Oral THC." *Clinical Chemistry, 55*(12), 2180–2189. https://doi.org/10.1373/clinchem.2008.122119

[332] Di Sabatino, A., Battista, N., Biancheri, P., Rapino, C., Rovedatti, L., Astarita, G., Vanoli, A., Dainese, E., Guerci, M., Piomelli, D., Pender, S. L., MacDonald, T. T., Maccarrone, M., & Corazza, G. R. (2011). "The endogenous cannabinoid system in the gut of patients with inflammatory bowel disease." *Mucosal Immunology, 4*(5), 574–583. https://doi.org/10.1038/mi.2011.18

[333] Wright, K. L., Rooney, N., Feeney, M., Tate, J. J. T., Robertson, D. R., Welham, M. J., & Ward, S. G. (2005). "Differential expression of cannabinoid receptors in the human colon: Cannabinoids promote epithelial wound healing." *Gastroenterology, 129*(2), 437–453. https://doi.org/10.1016/j.gastro.2005.05.026

[334] Di Sabatino, A., Battista, N., Biancheri, P., Rapino, C., Rovedatti, L., Astarita, G., Vanoli, A., Dainese, E., Guerci, M., Piomelli, D., Pender, S. L., MacDonald, T. T., Maccarrone, M., & Corazza, G. R. (2011). "The endogenous cannabinoid system in the gut of patients with inflammatory bowel disease." *Mucosal Immunology, 4*(5), 574–583. https://doi.org/10.1038/mi.2011.18

[335] Alhamoruni, A., Wright, K. L., Larvin, M., & O'Sullivan, S. E. (2012). "Cannabinoids mediate opposing effects on inflammation-induced intestinal permeability." *British Journal of Pharmacology, 165*(8), 2598–2610. https://doi.org/10.1111/j.1476-5381.2011.01589.x

Clinical studies that evaluated the effects of cannabis on Crohn's disease:

Study Type	Patient Sample Size	Treatment	Results	Reference
Retrospective observational study	30	Cannabis nonspecific treatment	Symptoms alleviation (HBI reduced from 14±6.7 to 7±4.7)	Stintzintzing et al., 2011
Prospective study	11	Cannabis use for 3 months	Symptoms alleviation (HBI reduced from 11.36±3.17 for 5.72±2.68)	Di Sabatino et al., 2011
Prospective study	21	115 mg of THC twice a day or placebo for 8 weeks	Remission (5/11), CDAI index reduction (10/11), quality of life increase	Singh et al., 2012
Prospective study	13	50 g cannabis per month (total 3 months)	Significant quality of life improvement, illness' activity and weight gain	Lahat; Lang; Shomron, 2012
Retrospective observational study	30	Orally or inhaled administered cannabis	Good clinical response (positive effect in disease' activity decreasing) and reduced need for other drugs and surgery	Naftali et al., 2011

Psoriasis

Psoriasis is a chronic inflammatory disease characterized by epidermal hyperplasia and inappropriate immune activation, which affects the skin and joints.[336,337,338] The exuberant epidermal alterations present in patients with psoriasis led physicians and researchers to guide treatments considering keratinocytes as the primary source of the alterations found in this disease. In 1977, it was demonstrated that the mononuclear inflammatory infiltration preceded the appearance of epidermal changes.[339] As early as 1978 and 1979, T lymphocytes and macrophages were identified as the predominant cells in dermal infiltration.[340] In addition, inflammatory infiltrates were phenotyped, and dendritic cells (DCs), macrophages, and CD4+ and CD8+ T lymphocytes were identified.[341]

Mast cells participate in inflammatory and allergic processes, collagen synthesis, immune reactions, tissue repair, neoplasms, and angiogenesis, and seem to be increased in psoriasis lesions. Inflammation is present in the psoriasis process due to the interaction of activated T lymphocytes with antigen-presenting cells and resident cells such as keratinocytes, synoviocytes, fibroblasts, and endothelial cells, which are in communication through cytokines, with TNF-α being the most important cytokine. The immune response mediated by T cells depends on their contact with DCs. Engagement of the T cell receptor (TCR) to the major histocompatibility complex (MHC) molecule on DCs sends the first signal that activates T cell proliferation, and sustaining this activation depends on the role of antigen-specific CD86 receptors on DCs. In addition, human leukocyte antigens (HLA) of classes I and II are essential in activating T lymphocytes during the immune response. The association of HLA molecules with the occurrence of psoriasis is described in the literature, and natural killer (NK) cells, effectors of innate immunity, have immunoglobulin-like receptors (KIR) on their

---

[336] Ryan, T. J. (1980). "Microcirculation in psoriasis: Blood vessels, lymphatics and tissue fluid." *Pharmacology & Therapeutics*, *10*(1), 27–64. https://doi.org/10.1016/0163-7258(80)90008-x

[337] Bull, R., Bates, D., & Mortimer, P. (1992). "Intravital video-capillaroscopy for the study of the microcirculation in psoriasis." *British Journal of Dermatology*, *126*(5), 436–445. https://doi.org/10.1111/j.1365-2133.1992.tb11815.x

[338] Boehncke, W., & Schön, M. P. (2007). "Animal models of psoriasis." *Clinics in Dermatology*, *25*(6), 596–605. https://doi.org/10.1016/j.clindermatol.2007.08.014

[339] Braun-Falco, O., & Schmoeckel, C. (1977). "The dermal inflammatory reaction in initial psoriatic lesions." *Archives of Dermatological Research*, *258*(1), 9–16. https://doi.org/10.1007/bf00582862

[340] Bjerke, J. R., & Krogh, H. (1978). "Identification of mononuclear cells in situ in skin lesions of lichen planus." *British Journal of Dermatology*, *98*(6), 605–610. https://doi.org/10.1111/j.1365-2133.1978.tb03577.x

[341] Bos, J. D., De Rie, M. A., Teunissen, M. B. M., & Pişkin, G. (2005). "Psoriasis: dysregulation of innate immunity." *British Journal of Dermatology*, *152*(6), 1098–1107. https://doi.org/10.1111/j.1365-2133.2005.06645.x

surface specific for class I HLA molecules, with an association reported of certain KIR and HLA-C alleles with increased susceptibility to psoriasis.[342]

Another factor related to pathological events in psoriasis is its relationship with the gut microbiome.[343] The gut microbiome in psoriasis cases is enriched with *Firmicutes* and *Actinobacteria spp.*, and its dysbiosis possibly causes metabolic alterations in the production and signaling of IL-23/IL-17 through the production of interferon-gamma (IFN-γ), leading to hyperproliferation of keratinocytes. The reduction of *Faecalibacterium prausnitzii* and *Akkermansia muciniphila* bacteria has been described in psoriasis,[344] and this type of bacteria is known to produce short-chain fatty acids and have anti-inflammatory actions.[345]

A schematic representation of the influence of the gut microbiota on psoriasis is shown below:

---

[342] Lowes, M. A., Suárez-Fariñas, M., & Krueger, J. G. (2014). "Immunology of psoriasis." *Annual Review of Immunology, 32*(1), 227–255. https://doi.org/10.1146/annurev-immunol-032713-120225

[343] Myers, B., Brownstone, N., Reddy, V., Chan, S., Thibodeaux, Q., Truong, A., Bhutani, T., Chang, H., & Liao, W. (2019). "The gut microbiome in psoriasis and psoriatic arthritis." *Best Practice & Research Clinical Rheumatology, 33*(6), 101494. https://doi.org/10.1016/j.berh.2020.101494

[344] Eppinga, H., Weiland, C. J. S., Thio, H. B., Van Der Woude, C. J., Nijsten, T., Peppelenbosch, M. P., & Konstantinov, S. R. (2016). "Similar Depletion of Protective *Faecalibacterium prausnitzii* in Psoriasis and Inflammatory Bowel Disease, but not in Hidradenitis Suppurativa." *Journal of Crohn's and Colitis, 10*(9), 1067–1075. https://doi.org/10.1093/ecco-jcc/jjw070

[345] Sitkin, S., & Pokrotnieks, J. (2018). "Clinical Potential of Anti-inflammatory Effects of *Faecalibacterium prausnitzii* and Butyrate in Inflammatory Bowel Disease." *Inflammatory Bowel Diseases, 25*(4), e40–e41. https://doi.org/10.1093/ibd/izy258

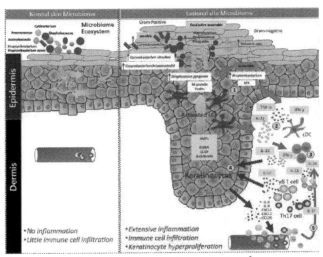
Gut microbiota and psoriasis.[346]

Phytocannabinoids & Psoriasis

The potential benefits of THC and CBD in therapy and regenerative medicine are shown by their regulatory effects on inflammation evidenced in *in vitro* and *in vivo* studies.[347,348] The study by Newton et al.[349] on the effects of THC on cells of the immune system showed that T cell activity can be suppressed with THC injections. In the study by Kusher et al.,[350] THC was able to regulate TNF-α and its formation in human lymphocytes.

Sangiovanni et al.[351] tested an extract of *Cannabis sativa* containing THC and CBD in human keratinocytes and fibroblasts. They demonstrated an

---

[346] Hsu, D. K., Fung, M. A., & Chen, H. (2020). Role of skin and gut microbiota in the pathogenesis of psoriasis, an inflammatory skin disease. *Medicine in Microecology, 4,* 100016. https://doi.org/10.1016/j.medmic.2020.100016

[347] Bos, J. D., De Rie, M. A., Teunissen, M. B. M., & Pişkin, G. (2005). "Psoriasis: dysregulation of innate immunity." *British Journal of Dermatology, 152*(6), 1098–1107. https://doi.org/10.1111/j.1365-2133.2005.06645.x

[348] Iffland, K., & Grotenhermen, F. (2017). "An update on safety and side effects of cannabidiol: a review of clinical data and relevant animal studies. *Cannabis and Cannabinoid Research, 2*(1), 139–154. https://doi.org/10.1089/can.2016.0034

[349] Shivers, S., Newton, C., Friedman, H., & Klein, T. (1994). "Δ9-tetrahydrocannabinol (THC) modulates IL-1 bioactivity in human monocyte/macrophage cell lines." *Life Sciences, 54*(17), 1281–1289. https://doi.org/10.1016/0024-3205(94)00856-6

[350] Kusher, D. I., Dawson, L. O., Taylor, A., & Djeu, J. Y. (1994). "Effect of the psychoactive metabolite of marijuana, Δ9-Tetrahydrocannabinol (THC), on the synthesis of tumor necrosis factor by human large granular lymphocytes." *Cellular Immunology, 154*(1), 99–108. https://doi.org/10.1006/cimm.1994.1060

[351] Sangiovanni E, Fumagalli M, Pacchetti B, Piazza S, Magnavacca A, Khalilpour S, Melzi G, Martinelli G, Dell'Agli M. "Cannabis sativa L. extract and cannabidiol inhibit in vitro mediators of skin inflammation and wound injury." *Phytother Res.* 2019 Aug;33(8):2083-2093. doi: 10.1002/ptr.6400. Epub 2019 Jun 27. PMID: 31250491.

inhibitory action on the activation of inflammatory factors mediated by NF-κB action. The results found in this study showed a decrease in the levels of IL-8, MMP-9, and VEGF, suggesting a therapeutic action on the skin. Furthermore, this study shows that the application of THC or CBD alone has different effects when compared to the combination of the two cannabinoids administered simultaneously.

There are few studies on the effects of cannabinoids on psoriasis in humans. In the study by Pacifici et al.,[352] blood samples from patients undergoing various levels of medical cannabis treatment were used, and levels of inflammatory markers were measured, as well as the lymphocyte activity of mitogens. A decrease in NK cell count, a decrease in lymphocyte proliferation, and IL-2 levels were observed, in addition to an increase in anti-inflammatory markers such as IL-10 and TGF-β1.

Angiogenesis, another psoriasis-involved mechanism, which consists of the formation of new blood vessels, is the target of psoriasis treatment, as demonstrated in the work of Heidenreich et al.,[353] and is divided into three distinct phases: proliferation, migration, and formation of endothelial cells. There is a correlation between HIF-1α and VEGF levels in the skin of patients with psoriasis.[354] Additionally, VEGF plasma levels may be associated with the severity of psoriasis.[355] In a clinical study, psoriasis patients with renal cancer were treated with bevacizumab, an anti-VEGF monoclonal antibody, and a complete remission of the disease was observed.[356]

As mentioned earlier, psoriasis has a direct relationship with inflammation and angiogenesis, and cannabinoids seem to have a therapeutic action in this

---

[352] Pacifici, R., Zuccaro, P., Pichini, S., Roset, P. N., Poudevida, S., Farré, M., Segura, J., & De La Torre, R. (2003). "Modulation of the immune system in cannabis users." *JAMA, 289*(15), 1929–1931. https://doi.org/10.1001/jama.289.15.1929-b

[353] Heidenreich, R., Röcken, M., & Ghoreschi, K. (2008). Angiogenesis: the new potential target for the therapy of psoriasis? *Drug News & Perspectives, 21*(2), 97. https://doi.org/10.1358/dnp.2008.21.2.1188196

[354] Simonetti, O., Lucarini, G., Goteri, G., Zizzi, A., Biagini, G., Lo Muzio, L., & Offidani, A. M. (2006) "Vegf is Likely a Key Factor in the Link between Inflammation and Angiogenesis in Psoriasis: Results of an Immunohistochemical Study." *International Journal of Immunopathology and Pharmacology, 19*(4), 751–760. https://doi.org/10.1177/039463200601900405

[355] Bhushan, M., McLaughlin, B., Weiss, J. B., & Griffiths, C. (1999). "Levels of endothelial cell stimulating angiogenesis factor and vascular endothelial growth factor are elevated in psoriasis." *British Journal of Dermatology, 141*(6), 1054–1060. https://doi.org/10.1046/j.1365-2133.1999.03205.x

[356] Datta-Mitra, A., Riar, N. K., & Raychaudhuri, S. P. (2014). "Remission of psoriasis and psoriatic arthritis during bevacizumab therapy for renal cell cancer." *Indian Journal of Dermatology, 59*(6), 632. https://doi.org/10.4103/0019-5154.143574

disease,[357] suppressing or inhibiting inflammatory processes and angiogenesis. JWH-133 is a selective synthetic cannabinoid and CB2 receptor agonist capable of inhibiting angiogenesis in *in vitro* studies.[358] A study by Blázquez et al.[359] demonstrated that after treatment with cannabinoids, endothelial cell proliferation decreased through the regulation of the expression of VEGF and the VEGFR-2 receptor.

In the study by Sugawara et al. with organoid culture and *knockout* mice for CB1 receptors, they investigated the inhibition of these receptors and how they can affect the biology of *in situ* cultures of epithelial tissues. The results of this study showed that the inhibition of CB1 receptors or the silencing of specific genes stimulates mast cell degranulation and maturation, showing that the *in situ* used model has good perspectives for the study of mast cell biology involving the effects of ECS.[360]

The study by Wilkinson and Williamson with cell culture of keratinocytes (since the inflammation of the disease is associated with the epithelial keratinocytes exacerbated proliferation) showed that isolated doses of THC, CBN, CBD, and CBG inhibited the proliferation of these cells in a dose-dependent manner, with a mean IC50 of 2.3 µM. When administered alone, these cannabinoids have been shown to have a similar effect on cell proliferation. The mechanism involved in explaining the results of this study consists in the fact that substances such as CBD were shown to be effective in inhibiting cell migration via the mediation of CB1-type receptors and the PPAR-γ receptor.[361]

---

[357] Norooznezhad, A. H., & Norooznezhad, F. (2017). "Cannabinoids: Possible agents for treatment of psoriasis via suppression of angiogenesis and inflammation." *Medical Hypotheses, 99*, 15–18. https://doi.org/10.1016/j.mehy.2016.12.003

[358] Vidinský B, Gál P, Pilátová M, et al. "Anti-proliferative and anti-angiogenic effects of CB2R agonist (JWH-133) in non-small lung cancer cells (A549) and human umbilical vein endothelial cells: an in vitro investigation." *Folia Biol (Praha).* 2012;58(2):75-80.

[359] Blázquez, C., González-Feria, L., Álvarez, L., Haro, A., Casanova, M., & Guzmán, M. (2004). "Cannabinoids inhibit the vascular endothelial growth factor pathway in gliomas." *Cancer Research, 64*(16), 5617–5623. https://doi.org/10.1158/0008-5472.can-03-3927

[360] Sugawara, K., BÍRó, T., Tsuruta, D., Tóth, B. I., Kromminga, A., Zákány, N., Zimmer, A., Funk, W., Gibbs, B. F., Zimmer, A., & Paus, R. (2012). "Endocannabinoids limit excessive mast cell maturation and activation in human skin." *The Journal of Allergy and Clinical Immunology, 129*(3), 726-738.e8. https://doi.org/10.1016/j.jaci.2011.11.009

[361] Wilkinson, J., & Williamson, E. M. (2007). "Cannabinoids inhibit human keratinocyte proliferation through a non-CB1/CB2 mechanism and have a potential therapeutic value in the treatment of psoriasis." *Journal of Dermatological Science, 45*(2), 87–92. https://doi.org/10.1016/j.jdermsci.2006.10.009

These works show the importance of endocannabinoids, mainly in the mechanisms involving cell proliferation and angiogenesis, which are commonly associated with inflammation. It can be seen that there is a scarcity of literature regarding clinical studies that prove the efficiency of cannabinoids, such as THC and CBD, in psoriasis treatment. In addition, the therapeutic perspectives shown in *in vitro* and *in vivo* studies are extremely important for Western medicine.

Multiple Sclerosis (MS)

The use of cannabinoids presents satisfactory therapeutic results and consistent evidence in the treatment of spasms and involuntary muscle contractions that usually evolve with pain and stiffness associated with MS. Clinical trials prove the safety and efficacy of drugs containing THC and CBD in improving the motor symptoms resulting from the disease. Several double-blind, randomized, placebo-controlled studies that followed participants diagnosed with MS demonstrated by different analysis methodologies that treatment with cannabinoids was able to significantly and safely reduce spasms.[362,363,364,365,366] A meta-analysis study considered a moderate-quality degree of evidence regarding the treatment of spasticity with cannabinoids.[367] In 2017, Mevatyl®, an oral spray containing THC and CBD in the same proportion, was registered as the first cannabis-based

---

[362] Collin, C., Davies, P., Mutiboko, I. K., & Ratcliffe, S. (2007). "Randomized controlled trial of cannabis-based medicine in spasticity caused by multiple sclerosis." *European Journal of Neurology, 14*(3), 290–296. https://doi.org/10.1111/j.1468-1331.2006.01639.x

[363] Novotná, A., Mares, J., Ratcliffe, S., Nováková, I., Vachová, M., Zapletalová, O., Gasperini, C., Pozzilli, C., Cefaro, L. A., Comi, G., Rossi, P., Ambler, Z., Stelmasiak, Z., Erdmann, A., Montalbán, X., Klimek, A., & Davies, P. (2011). "A randomized, double-blind, placebo-controlled, parallel-group, enriched-design study of nabiximols* (Sativex®), as add-on therapy, in subjects with refractory spasticity caused by multiple sclerosis." *European Journal of Neurology, 18*(9), 1122–1131. https://doi.org/10.1111/j.1468-1331.2010.03328.x

[364] Patti, F., Messina, S., Solaro, C., Amato, M. P., Bergamaschi, R., Bonavita, S., Bossio, R. B., Morra, V. B., Costantino, G., Cavalla, P., Centonze, D., Comi, G., Cottone, S., Danni, M., Francia, A., Gajofatto, A., Gasperini, C., Ghezzi, A., Iudice, A., ... Zappia, M. (2016). "Efficacy and safety of cannabinoid oromucosal spray for multiple sclerosis spasticity." *Journal of Neurology, Neurosurgery, and Psychiatry, 87*(9), 944–951. https://doi.org/10.1136/jnnp-2015-312591

[365] Zettl, U. K., Rommer, P., Hipp, P., & Patejdl, R. (2015). "Evidence for the efficacy and effectiveness of THC-CBD oromucosal spray in symptom management of patients with spasticity due to multiple sclerosis." *Therapeutic Advances in Neurological Disorders, 9*(1), 9–30. https://doi.org/10.1177/1756285615612659

[366] Marková, J., Essner, U., Akmaz, B., Marinelli, M., Trompke, C., Lentschat, A., & Vila, C. (2018). "Sativex® as add-on therapy vs. further optimized first-line ANTispastics (SAVANT) in resistant multiple sclerosis spasticity: a double-blind, placebo-controlled randomised clinical trial." *International Journal of Neuroscience, 129*(2), 119–128. https://doi.org/10.1080/00207454.2018.1481066

[367] Whiting, P., Wolff, R., Deshpande, S., Di Nisio, M., Duffy, S., Hernández, A. V., Keurentjes, J. C., Lang, S., Misso, K., Ryder, S., Schmidlkofer, S., Westwood, M., & Kleijnen, J. (2015). "Cannabinoids for medical use." *JAMA, 313*(24), 2456. https://doi.org/10.1001/jama.2015.6358

herbal medicine in Brazil, registered in 28 countries under the name of Sativex®, and indicated for reducing MS spasms.

Cancer & Symptoms Arising from its Treatment

Anecdotal stories and scientific research have ignited interest in the use of cannabinoids for cancer treatment. In a March 17, 2011 update, the US National Cancer Institute (NCI) addressed the relationship between cancer treatment and cannabis. This update was censored and removed just 11 days after its initial release. The Institute acknowledged that "the potential effects of medicinal cannabis for people living with cancer include antiemetic effects, appetite stimulation, pain relief, anxiolytic, and sleep improvement. In the practice of oncology integration, the health professional may recommend medicinal cannabis not only for symptom management but also for a possible direct antitumor effect."

NCI followed this release with new information and a report that implied a connection between smoking, as opposed to oral ingestion of cannabis, and an increased risk of lung and certain digestive system cancers. This "fake news" led to an intense backlash from Advocates for the Disabled and Seriously Ill (ADSI). According to ADSI, the results of 19 government studies failed to "demonstrate statistically significant associations between cannabis inhalation and lung cancer." The report also identified a separate study of 611 patients with lung cancer that showed that cannabis "is not associated with an increased risk of lung cancer or other upper aerodigestive tract cancers and found no positive associations with any cancer type."[368] The ADSI further noted a study by Spanish researcher Dr. Manuel Guzmán on synthetic THC (dronabinol), in which patients with recurrent glioblastoma were given an intratumoral injection of Δ^9-THC. The study resulted in tumor reduction in several test participants.[369]

One of the main ways that cannabinoids appear to act in cancer is by promoting apoptosis. Endocannabinoids can create a positive feedback loop, increasing stress to the point where the cancer cell self-destructs.[370]

---

[368] Huang YH, Zhang ZF, Tashkin DP, Feng B, Straif K, Hashibe M. "An epidemiologic review of marijuana and cancer: an update." *Cancer Epidemiol Biomarkers.* Prev. 2015 Jan. 24 (1):15-31. doi: 10.1158/1055-9965.EPI-14-1026. PMID: 25587109; PMCID: PMC4302404.

[369] *Ibid.*

[370] Ligresti, A., De Petrocellis, L., & Di Marzo, V. (2016b). "From phytocannabinoids to cannabinoid receptors and endocannabinoids: pleiotropic physiological and pathological roles through complex pharmacology". *Physiological Reviews,* 96(4), 1593–1659. https://doi.org/10.1152/physrev.00002.2016

Phytocannabinoids can also induce apoptosis under similar conditions. The death of cancer cells promotes homeostasis and survival of the organism.

Researchers in Great Britain found that *in vivo* cancer cells contain cannabinoid receptors on the surface of the cell wall. The introduction of exogenous cannabinoids to cancer cells induced apoptosis of only the cancer cell. The presence of cannabinoids also prohibits the production of angiogenic growth factor (AGF) from cancer cells. This growth factor is utilized by cancer cells to develop their own blood supply. It is a reasonable assumption to conclude that without a blood supply, cancer cells cannot proliferate.[371]

Researchers in Israel have also studied the effectiveness of cannabis in inhibiting cancer. This research is well-elucidated in Dr. Joe Goldstrich's book *The Cannabis Cancer Connection* (2023).[372]

A report by British researchers in the *Journal of Neuroscience* noted that "under pathological conditions, in relation to mitochondrial dysfunction and calcium dysregulation, CBD may prove beneficial in promoting apoptotic signaling through restoration of calcium homeostasis."[373] CBD regulates the ebb and flow of calcium and stress, autophagy and cell death, and restores homeostasis at a cellular level. Further evidence of the ability of cannabis to promote apoptosis of cancer cells and the inhibition of the ability of cancer cells to emit angiogenic growth factor (AGF).[374]

In vitro studies performed by GW Pharmaceuticals have determined that the phytocannabinoids CBN, CBD, and CBG are effective in inhibiting aggressive cancers.[375] They found that a synergistic increase in antiproliferative and apoptotic (cell-killing) activity of cannabinoids can be produced by combining specific ratios of CB1 and CB2 receptor agonists with non-

---

[371] Guzman, M. "Cannabinoids as Possible Antitumoral Drugs." Presented at the Tenth National Clinical Conference on Cannabis Therapeutics.; 2016; Baltimore,, MD.

[372] Goldstrich, J. D. (2023). *The Cannabis Cancer Connection: How to use cannabis and hemp to kill cancer cells*. Flower Valley Press.

[373] Ryan, D., Drysdale, A. J., Lafourcade, C., Pertwee, R. G., & Platt, B. (2009). "Cannabidiol Targets Mitochondria to Regulate Intracellular Ca2+Levels." *The Journal of Neuroscience*, 29(7), 2053–2063. https://doi.org/10.1523/jneurosci.4212-08.2009

[374] Werner, C. (2011). *Marijuana: Gateway to health: How cannabis protects us from cancer and Alzheimers disease*. San Francisco: Dachstar Press.

[375] Velasco, G., Sánchez, C., & Guzmán, M. (2016). "Anticancer mechanisms of cannabinoids." *Current Oncology*, 23(11), 23–32. https://doi.org/10.3747/co.23.3080

psychotropic cannabinoids.[376] In 2019, GW completed a glioblastoma study using a full-spectrum cannabis alcohol extract containing 25 mg of THC and 25 mg of CBD three times a day. The study group experienced an 83% one-year survival rate compared to a 53% one-year survival rate for those with conventional treatment alone.

In addition to phytocannabinoids, terpenes also play a role in apoptosis. M. N. Gould describes this process: "Monoterpenes are found in the essential oil of many plants, including fruits, vegetables, and herbs [and] impede the process of carcinogenesis in both the early and promotion/progression stages." Furthermore, monoterpenes are effective in treating early and advanced cancers by inhibiting isoprenylation of small G proteins, which can alter signal transduction and result in altered gene expression.[377]

In animal models, these compounds have shown efficacy in treating several cancers, including breast and pancreatic carcinomas. Furthermore, *in vitro* data suggest they may effectively treat neuroblastomas and leukemias. Both limonene and Perillyl alcohol (a terpene found in lavender and lemongrass) are being evaluated in clinical trials in patients with advanced cancer.[378]

Symptoms Caused by Chemotherapy Treatments

One of the first uses of cannabinoids for proven therapeutic purposes in contemporary times was the reduction of nausea and vomiting triggered by chemotherapy. A meta-analysis evaluating 30 randomized clinical trials from 1975 to 1996 indicated that cannabinoids were more effective than placebo and completely stopped chemotherapy-induced nausea and vomiting in all assessed studies. Control groups in these trials ranged from placebos to active drugs indicated for this purpose. These findings were corroborated by another meta-analysis study that proved the antiemetic effect of cannabinoids associated with therapies for the treatment of cancer.[379]

---

[376] Plc, G. P. (2017, February 7). "GW Pharmaceuticals achieves positive results in Phase 2 proof of concept study in Glioma." *GlobeNewswire News Room.* https://www.globenewswire.com/news-release/2017/02/07/914583/0/en/GW-Pharmaceuticals-Achieves-Positive-Results-in-Phase-2-Proof-of-Concept-Study-in-Glioma.html

[377] Gould, M. N. (1997). "Cancer chemoprevention and therapy by monoterpenes." *Environmental Health Perspectives, 105*(suppl 4), 977–979. https://doi.org/10.1289/ehp.97105s4977

[378] Belville, R. (2017, December 7). "National Cancer Institute scrubs 'Antitumoral effect' of cannabinoids from website." *HuffPost.* http://www.huffingtonpost.com/russ-belville/national-cancer-institute_b_842631.html/

[379] Rocha, F. R., Stefano, S. C., De Cássia Haiek, R., Oliveira, L., & Da Silveira, D. X. (2008). "Therapeutic use of *Cannabis sativa* on chemotherapy-induced nausea and vomiting among cancer patients: systematic

Another meta-analysis confirmed the efficacy and safety of this treatment. It highlights that although there is evidence of effectiveness, most of the studies are old, and comparisons with new chemotherapies and new antiemetic agents should be performed to confirm whether this treatment overcomes the effects of these new classes of drugs.[380]

Neurodegenerative & Neurodevelopment-Related Diseases

The stories of children with intractable (untreatable) epilepsy who experienced incredible medical success with high-CBD cannabis propelled the use of medical cannabis into the mainstream and is largely responsible for medical professionals worldwide taking a closer look. It is now known that cannabis has the potential to treat or mitigate the symptoms of many neurodegenerative or neurodevelopment-related diseases.

A study published in the *Journal of Neuroscience* demonstrated that synthetic cannabinoids could be successful in preventing neurodegenerative processes, a finding likely associated with the fact that cannabinoids are neuroprotective and can prevent neuronal cell death.[381] This study is one of many that suggest that cannabinoids can treat inflammation in the brain and may protect humans from the cognitive decline associated with, for example, Alzheimer's disease.

As interest in the use of cannabis to treat epilepsy has grown, so has research and demand for it to treat other neurodegenerative and neurodevelopment-related disorders, particularly autism and Alzheimer's disease. Cannabis is now being used to treat autism, particularly in children with very severe symptoms. It also holds great promise for treating Alzheimer's. This chapter takes a closer look at the available research surrounding these conditions.

---

review and meta-analysis." *European Journal of Cancer Care, 17*(5), 431–443. https://doi.org/10.1111/j.1365-2354.2008.00917.x

[380] Smith, L. A., Azariah, F., Lavender, V., Stoner, N., & Bettiol, S. (2015). "Cannabinoids for nausea and vomiting in adults with cancer receiving chemotherapy." *The Cochrane Library, 2021*(11). https://doi.org/10.1002/14651858.cd009464.pub2

[381] Ramírez, B. G., Blázquez, C., Del Pulgar, T. G., Guzmán, M., & De Ceballos, M. L. (n.d.). "Prevention of Alzheimer's Disease Pathology by Cannabinoids: Neuroprotection Mediated by Blockade of Microglial Activation." *The Journal of Neuroscience.* https://doi.org/10.1523/jneurosci.4540-04.2005

Epilepsy

The most robust evidence for the cannabinoids' therapeutic use is for conventional treatment-resistant epilepsy. In 1843, the first case report was published on the use of cannabis tincture for the remission of seizures in a 40-day-old child.[382] The case was reported by William O'Shaughnessy, an Irish physician who lived in India, where cannabis use is traditional.

The first placebo-controlled clinical trial involving epileptic individuals being treated with phytocannabinoids was carried out in Brazil by Prof. Elisaldo Carlini. In this study, eight patients were treated with about 200 mg/day of CBD; of these patients, four had seizures completely abolished, while another three had a significant reduction in seizure frequency. Only one participant did not show improvement.[383] Recently, clinical studies have been published in prestigious and accredited medical journals aimed to evaluate the effectiveness and safety of CBD treatments in people diagnosed with rare genetic syndromes such as Dravet and Lennox-Gastaut. These diseases cause, among other symptoms, epileptic encephalopathy. There was a significant reduction in the frequency of seizures in participants in both studies. CBD can be pointed out as an important adjuvant to conventional treatments with anticonvulsants, especially in the pediatric population resistant to conventional treatments.[384,385,386] A systematic review on the subject points out that high-quality clinical trials show the possibility of treatment using CBD for resistant epilepsy in pediatrics; however, it emphasizes that this finding was limited to CBD and cannot be extended to

---

[382] O'Shaughnessy WB. "On the preparations of the Indian Hemp, or Gunjah: Cannabis indica their effects on the animal system in health, and their utility in the treatment of tetanus and other convulsive diseases." Prov Med J Retrosp Med Sci. 1843;5(123):363-369.

[383] Cunha, J. M., Carlini, E. A., Pereira, A. E., Ramos, O. L., Pimentel, C., Gagliardi, R. J., Sanvito, W. L., Lander, N., & Mechoulam, R. (1980). "Chronic administration of cannabidiol to healthy volunteers and epileptic patients." *Pharmacology, 21*(3), 175–185. https://doi.org/10.1159/000137430

[384] Devinsky, O., Cross, J. H., Laux, L., Marsh, E. D., Miller, I., Nabbout, R., Scheffer, I. E., Thiele, E. A., & Wright, S. (2017). "Trial of cannabidiol for Drug-Resistant seizures in the Dravet Syndrome." *The New England Journal of Medicine, 376*(21), 2011–2020. https://doi.org/10.1056/nejmoa1611618

[385] Thiele, E. A., Marsh, E. D., French, J. A., Mazurkiewicz-Bełdzińska, M., Benbadis, S. R., Joshi, C., Lyons, P. D., Taylor, A., Roberts, C., Sommerville, K. W., Gunning, B., Gawłowicz, J., Lisewski, P., Beldzinska, M. M., Szewczyk, K., Steinborn, B., Żołnowska, M., Hughes, E., McLellan, A., ... Wilfong, A. A. (2018). "Cannabidiol in patients with seizures associated with Lennox-Gastaut syndrome (GWPCARE4): a randomised, double-blind, placebo-controlled phase 3 trial." *The Lancet, 391*(10125), 1085–1096. https://doi.org/10.1016/s0140-6736(18)30136-3

[386] Devinsky, O., Verducci, C., Thiele, E. A., Laux, L., Patel, A. D., Filloux, F., Szaflarski, J. P., Wilfong, A. A., Clark, G. D., Park, Y. D., Seltzer, L. E., Bebin, E. M., Flamini, R., Wechsler, R., & Friedman, D. (2018). "Open-label use of highly purified CBD (Epidiolex®) in patients with CDKL5 deficiency disorder and Aicardi, Dup15q, and Doose syndromes." *Epilepsy & Behavior, 86*, 131–137. https://doi.org/10.1016/j.yebeh.2018.05.013

other cannabis-based products.[387] A meta-analysis study demonstrates that extracts enriched with CBD had a better result in reducing the frequency of seizures, with a lower dose and fewer adverse events when compared to studies that evaluated the use of CBD alone.[388]

Autism

Autism Spectrum Disorders (ASD) are a group of complex neurological disorders whose clinical manifestations are generally characterized by functional deficits in three areas: mental development, social interaction, and behavior,[389] with an estimated worldwide prevalence of 62 in 10,000.[390,391] According to the criteria of the Diagnostic Manual of Mental Disorders (DSM-5), these disorders can be divided into Asperger's Syndrome, characterized by delayed verbal communication and impaired cognitive development; typical autism, characterized by alterations in the three main behavioral domains and evidenced before the age of three years; and pervasive developmental disorders not otherwise specified.[392]

The clinical manifestations present in ASD include changes in sensory sensitivity, attention deficit, hyperactivity, anxiety, gastrointestinal complications, increased susceptibility to seizures and epileptic seizures, intellectual disability, and self-injurious behavior.[393] Some pathological manifestations present in patients with ASD are observed, for example, through neuroanatomical alterations detected by magnetic resonance

---

[387] Elliott, J., DeJean, D., Clifford, T., Coyle, D., Potter, B. K., Skidmore, B., Alexander, C., Repetski, A. E., Shukla, V. K., McCoy, B., & Wells, G. A. (2018). "Cannabis-based products for pediatric epilepsy: A systematic review." *Epilepsia*, 60(1), 6–19. https://doi.org/10.1111/epi.14608

[388] Pamplona, F. A., Da Silva, L. R., & Coan, A. C. (2018). "Potential Clinical Benefits of CBD-Rich cannabis extracts over Purified CBD in Treatment-Resistant Epilepsy: Observational Data Meta-analysis." *Frontiers in Neurology*, 9. https://doi.org/10.3389/fneur.2018.00759

[389] American Psychiatric Association. *Diagnostic and Statistical Manual of Mental Disorders*. 5th ed. Washington D.C., 2013

[390] Elsabbagh, M., Divan, G., Koh, Y. J., Kim, Y. S., Kauchali, S., Marcín, C., Montiel-Nava, C., Patel, V., De Paula, C. S., Wang, C., Yasamy, M. T., & Fombonne, É. (2012). "Global prevalence of autism and other pervasive developmental disorders." *Autism Research*, 5(3), 160–179. https://doi.org/10.1002/aur.239

[391] Fleury-Teixeira, P., Caixeta, F. V., Da Silva, L. C. R., Brasil–Neto, J. P., & Malcher-Lopes, R. (2019). "Effects of CBD-Enriched Cannabis sativa Extract on Autism Spectrum Disorder Symptoms: An Observational Study of 18 Participants Undergoing Compassionate Use." *Frontiers in Neurology*, 10. https://doi.org/10.3389/fneur.2019.01145

[392] Lai, W. W., & Oei, T. P. S. (2014). "Coping in Parents and Caregivers of Children with Autism Spectrum Disorders (ASD): a Review." *Review Journal of Autism and Developmental Disorders*, 1(3), 207–224. https://doi.org/10.1007/s40489-014-0021-x

[393] Lord, C., Cook, E. H., Leventhal, B. L., & Amaral, D. G. (2000). "Autism spectrum disorders." *Neuron*, 28(2), 355–363. https://doi.org/10.1016/s0896-6273(00)00115-x

imaging, such as changes in the size of the cerebellum, hippocampus, and amygdala. However, these changes are not usually associated with ASD because they are present in other more common neurological disorders.[394] It is believed that the changes observed in ASD have multifactorial causes, but are generally found to be associated with chromosomal mutations or epigenetic changes in different genes, often associated with neuronal functions.[395] Thus, ASD can be considered a disease with greater genetic repercussions when compared to pathophysiological origins, in line with a previous study that estimated 80–90% heritability for ASD.[396]

Some works, such as Vortsman et al. and Xu et al.[397,398] were made in an attempt to clarify the cause of ASD in different chromosomal and gene regions. However, in the work of Kusenda and Sebat,[399] chromosomal abnormalities were identified in the regions 15q11-13, 16p11.2, and 22q11.3 with greater frequency in patients diagnosed with ASD. In addition to the work of Kusenda and Sebat, other genes were identified, such as the RELN gene, which is involved in the regulation of synaptic plasticity and the release of neurotransmitters in the nervous system,[400,401] as well as others such as

---

[394] Rubenstein, J. L., & Merzenich, M. M. (2003). "Model of autism: increased ratio of excitation/inhibition in key neural systems." *Genes, Brain and Behavior*, 2(5), 255–267. https://doi.org/10.1034/j.1601-183x.2003.00037.x

[395] Schroeder, J. C., Reim, D., Boeckers, T. M., & Schmeißer, M. J. (2015). "Genetic animal models for autism spectrum disorder." In *Current topics in behavioral neurosciences* (pp. 311–324). https://doi.org/10.1007/7854_2015_407

[396] Muhle, R., Trentacoste, S., & Rapin, I. (2004). "The genetics of autism." *Pediatrics*, 113(5), e472–e486. https://doi.org/10.1542/peds.113.5.e472

[397] Vorstman, J., Staal, W., Hochstenbach, P. F. R., Franke, L., Van Daalen, E., & Van Engeland, H. (2005). "Overview of cytogenetic regions of interest (CROIs) associated with the autism phenotype across the human genome." *Molecular Psychiatry*, 11(1), 1. https://doi.org/10.1038/sj.mp.4001781

[398] Xu, L., Li, J. R., Huang, Y., Zhao, M., Tang, X., & Wei, L. (2011). "AutismKB: an evidence-based knowledgebase of autism genetics." *Nucleic Acids Research*, 40(D1), D1016–D1022. https://doi.org/10.1093/nar/gkr1145

[399] Kusenda, M., & Sebat, J. (2008). "The role of rare structural variants in the genetics of autism spectrum disorders." *Cytogenetic and Genome Research*, 123(1–4), 36–43. https://doi.org/10.1159/000184690

[400] Xu, L., Li, J. R., Huang, Y., Zhao, M., Tang, X., & Wei, L. (2011b). "AutismKB: an evidence-based knowledgebase of autism genetics." *Nucleic Acids Research*, 40(D1), D1016–D1022. https://doi.org/10.1093/nar/gkr1145

[401] Persico, A. M., D'Agruma, L., Maiorano, N., Totaro, A., Militerni, R., Bravaccio, C., Wassink, T. H., Schneider, C., Melmed, R. D., Trillo, S., Montecchi, F., Palermo, M. T., Pascucci, T., Puglisi-Allegra, S., Reichelt, K. L., Conciatori, M., Marino, R., Quattrocchi, C. C., Baldi, A., ... Keller, F. (2001). "Reelin gene alleles and haplotypes as a factor predisposing to autistic disorder." *Molecular Psychiatry*, 6(2), 150–159. https://doi.org/10.1038/sj.mp.4000850

neuroligin 3 and 4 (NLGN 3 and NLGN4),[402] neurexin 1 (NRXN1)[403] and SHANK3 (SH3 and multiple ankyrin repeat domains 3),[404] commonly related to synaptic maturation and which are more frequent in patients with ASD. Another study showed a susceptibility in genes related to ASD in three biological pathways activated by BDNF/TrkB, such as changes in the expression of the gene encoding the neurotrophic receptor tyrosine kinase 2 (NTRK2) and the genes participating in the PI3K/Akt pathway.[405]

There is great genetic heterogeneity in patients with ASD, and some genetic models have been suggested to explain the genetic variability present in autism, highlighting the multifactorial model of inheritance, which involves the combination of allelic variants added to each other or to environmental factors; models involving two or more genes (two-hit or multi-hit); and the single gene model of inheritance.[406] For a better understanding of genetic heterogeneity, these genes are associated with common molecular pathways that are related to the control of protein synthesis at synapses, such as the intracellular signaling pathway PI3K-mTOR (phosphatidylinositol-3-kinase-mammalian target of rapamycin).[407]

Currently, there are no drugs or other psychotherapeutic approaches capable of significantly improving the quality of life, social skills, and cognitive development in patients with more severe ASD.[408] Antipsychotic, antidepressant, antiepileptic, or anxiolytic drugs can improve the aggressive

---

[402] Jamain, S., Quach, H., Betancur, C., Råstam, M., Colineaux, C., Gillberg, I. C., Söderström, H., Giros, B., Leboyer, M., Gillberg, C., & Bourgeron, T. (2003). "Mutations of the X-linked genes encoding neuroligins NLGN3 and NLGN4 are associated with autism." *Nature Genetics*, 34(1), 27–29. https://doi.org/10.1038/ng1136

[403] Vicente, A. M. (2010). *Envolvimento da via de sinalização BNDF/TRKB na etiologia do autismo: análise genética*. http://hdl.handle.net/10451/2412

[404] Durand, C., Betancur, C., Boeckers, T. M., Bockmann, J., Chaste, P., Fauchereau, F., Nygren, G., Råstam, M., Gillberg, I. C., Anckarsäter, H., Sponheim, E., Goubran-Botros, H., Delorme, R., Chabane, N., Mouren-Siméoni, M., De Mas, P., Bieth, É., Rogé, B., Héron, D., ... Bourgeron, T. (2006). "Mutations in the gene encoding the synaptic scaffolding protein SHANK3 are associated with autism spectrum disorders." *Nature Genetics*, 39(1), 25–27. https://doi.org/10.1038/ng1933

[405] Vicente, A. M. (2010d). *Envolvimento da via de sinalização BNDF/TRKB na etiologia do autismo: análise genética*. http://hdl.handle.net/10451/2412

[406] El-Fishawy, P., & State, M. W. (2010). "The Genetics of Autism: key issues, recent findings, and clinical implications." *Psychiatric Clinics of North America*, 33(1), 83–105. https://doi.org/10.1016/j.psc.2009.12.002

[407] Kelleher, R. J., & Bear, M. F. (2008). "The autistic Neuron: troubled translation?" *Cell*, 135(3), 401–406. https://doi.org/10.1016/j.cell.2008.10.017

[408] Fleury-Teixeira, P., Caixeta, F. V., Da Silva, L. C. R., Brasil-Neto, J. P., & Malcher-Lopes, R. (2019b). "Effects of CBD-Enriched Cannabis sativa Extract on Autism Spectrum Disorder Symptoms: An Observational Study of 18 Participants Undergoing Compassionate Use." *Frontiers in Neurology*, 10. https://doi.org/10.3389/fneur.2019.01145

behavior of these patients, among other positive effects on behavior. However, the side effects of these drugs are sometimes greater than the beneficial effects, in addition to not contributing to aspects related to social interaction, which have a great impact on the daily lives of patients and their families.[409]

Phytocannabinoids and Autism

The endocannabinoid system (ECS) is commonly affected in patients with ASD. One of the mechanisms involved is the interaction between signaling and oxytocin mediators. Wei et al. showed that oxytocin, a neuropeptide that is related to strengthening social and parental bonds, mobilizes anandamide (AEA, the endocannabinoid analog of THC) in the nucleus accumbens (NAc) of rats. This study showed that AEA signaling at CB1 receptors (mediated by oxytocin) modulates social responses and that AEA deficits may contribute to social interaction effects in patients with ASD.[410] Corroborating these data sets, the study by Anagnostou et al.[411] demonstrated that the oral and daily administration of oxytocin can promote therapeutic effects in patients with ASD, as it leads to the improvement of functional and cognitive deficits and repetitive movements.

The administration of cannabinoids to children and adolescents is controversial in scientific literature due to the suspicion that it can influence brain development, consisting of maturation processes and rearrangements, such as myelination and synaptic plasticity, in addition to the maturation of neurotransmitter systems, as well as the ECS.[412] The ECS is commonly found to be altered in patients with ASD when related to comorbidities such as sequelae, anxiety, and cognitive and sleep disorders. A 2018 study even showed that AEA signaling may be involved in the pathophysiology of ASD.[413]

---

[409] IJff, D. M., & Aldenkamp, A. P. (2013). "Cognitive side-effects of antiepileptic drugs in children." In *Handbook of Clinical Neurology* (pp. 707–718). https://doi.org/10.1016/b978-0-444-52891-9.00073-7

[410] Wei, X., Christiano, E. R. A., Yu, J., Wagner, M., & Spiker, D. (2014). "Reading and math achievement profiles and longitudinal growth trajectories of children with an autism spectrum disorder." *Autism, 19*(2), 200–210. https://doi.org/10.1177/1362361313516549

[411] Anagnostou, E., & Taylor, M. J. (2011). "Review of neuroimaging in autism spectrum disorders: what have we learned and where do we go from here." *Molecular Autism, 2*(1), 4. https://doi.org/10.1186/2040-2392-2-4

[412] Chakrabarti, B., Persico, A. M., Battista, N., & Maccarrone, M. (2015). "Endocannabinoid signaling in autism." *Neurotherapeutics, 12*(4), 837–847. https://doi.org/10.1007/s13311-015-0371-9

[413] Karhson, D. S., Krasinska, K., Ahloy-Dallaire, J., Libove, R. A., Phillips, J. M., Chien, A., Garner, J. P., Hardan, A. Y., & Parker, K. J. (2018). "Plasma anandamide concentrations are lower in children with autism spectrum disorder." *Molecular Autism, 9*(1). https://doi.org/10.1186/s13229-018-0203-y

Observational studies and case reports have identified a possible therapeutic potential of phytocannabinoids from the use of pure CBD or CBD integrated with THC in the treatment of autism.[414,415,416] Such studies, which included the use of CBD and THC extracts in a 20:1 ratio, showed that in children and adolescents, the side effects of these compounds are lower when compared to those of drugs traditionally prescribed for the treatment of autism and epilepsy.[417]

The epidemiological study by Bar-Lev Schleider et al.[418] involved data from 188 patients with autism treated with oil composed of 30% CBD and 1.5% THC between 2015 and 2017. The results showed that after six months, 82.4% of the patients (155) were actively undergoing treatment, and, of these, 60% (93) were assessed globally. Of the total evaluated, 28 patients (30.1%) reported significant improvement in symptoms; 50 patients (53.7%) reported moderate improvement; six patients (6.4%) reported small improvement; and eight patients (8.6%) had no change in their health status. In general, the use of cannabis was well-tolerated since only 6.6% of the patients reported some degree of restlessness, and most of them showed improvement in the symptoms associated with autism.

In a retrospective study by Aran et al.[419] involving 60 children aged 11.8±3.5 years with ASD and severe behavioral problems, an extract containing CBD and THC in a 20:1 ratio, infused in olive oil, was administered two to three times a day for 2-4 weeks. The researchers observed improvement in 61% of behavioral changes and found that, at high doses, psychotic events can be triggered. In this sense, other studies have also shown that CBD treatment

---

[414] O'Connell, B. K., Gloss, D., & Devinsky, O. (2017). "Cannabinoids in treatment-resistant epilepsy: A review." *Epilepsy & Behavior, 70*, 341–348. https://doi.org/10.1016/j.yebeh.2016.11.012

[415] Ridler, C. (2017). "Cannabidiol reduces seizure frequency in Dravet syndrome." *Nature Reviews Neurology, 13*(7), 383. https://doi.org/10.1038/nrneurol.2017.86

[416] Rosenberg, E. C., Louik, J., Conway, E., Devinsky, O., & Friedman, D. J. (2017). "Quality of Life in Childhood Epilepsy in pediatric patients enrolled in a prospective, open-label clinical study with cannabidiol." *Epilepsia, 58*(8), e96–e100. https://doi.org/10.1111/epi.13815

[417] Lai, W. W., & Oei, T. P. S. (2014b). "Coping in Parents and Caregivers of Children with Autism Spectrum Disorders (ASD): a Review." *Review Journal of Autism and Developmental Disorders, 1*(3), 207–224. https://doi.org/10.1007/s40489-014-0021-x

[418] Schleider, L. B., Mechoulam, R., Saban, N., Meiri, G., & Novack, V. (2019). "Real life Experience of Medical Cannabis Treatment in Autism: Analysis of Safety and Efficacy." *Scientific Reports, 9*(1). https://doi.org/10.1038/s41598-018-37570-y

[419] Aran, A., Cassuto, H., Lubotzky, A., Wattad, N., & Hazan, E. (2018). "Brief Report: Cannabidiol-Rich Cannabis in Children with Autism Spectrum Disorder and Severe Behavioral Problems—A Retrospective Feasibility Study." *Journal of Autism and Developmental Disorders, 49*(3), 1284–1288. https://doi.org/10.1007/s10803-018-3808-2

improved autism spectrum disorder-related symptoms such as anger, self-injury, hyperactivity, sleep problems, and anxiety.[420,421]

In an observational cohort study, 18 autistic patients were treated with manufactured CBD containing approximately 75:1 CBD/THC, administered in capsules containing 25 or 50 mg CBD and 0.34 mg or 0.68 mg THC, respectively. After six to nine months of treatment, improvement in symptoms such as attention deficit, hyperactivity, sleep disorders, and improvement in social communication was observed.[422] Still in clinical studies, Barchel et al. observed controversial results.[423] Fifty-three children with ASD were evaluated, with a mean age of 11 years (4-22), who were treated with CBD-rich oil tablets for about 66 days. Of the total number of patients, 67.6% presented self-harm; 68.4% had hyperactivity; 71.4% had sleep disorders; and 47.1% developed anxiety, representing the worsening of the autism case.

Another strand of studies on autism shows the action of neuroligins, which are postsynaptic cell adhesion molecules expressed in four main isoforms (neuroligins 1-4; NL1-NL4).[424] In humans, more than 30 neuroligin gene mutations have been linked to autism, especially NL3, which is found at both excitatory and inhibitory synapses. According to the study by Földy et al, NL3 is essential for the tonic signaling of the ECS, and mice with an NL3 mutation (R451C), which mimics autism in humans, develop important synaptic alterations involving the somatosensory cortex and the hippocampus.[425]

---

[420] Barchel, D., Stolar, O., De-Haan, T., Ziv-Baran, T., Saban, N., Fuchs, D. O., Koren, G., & Berkovitch, M. (2019). "Oral cannabidiol use in children with autism spectrum disorder to treat related symptoms and co-morbidities." *Frontiers in Pharmacology*, 9. https://doi.org/10.3389/fphar.2018.01521

[421] Poleg, S., Golubchik, P., Offen, D., & Weizman, A. (2019). "Cannabidiol as a suggested candidate for treatment of autism spectrum disorder." *Progress in Neuro-Psychopharmacology and Biological Psychiatry*, 89, 90–96. https://doi.org/10.1016/j.pnpbp.2018.08.030

[422] Lai, W. W., & Oei, T. P. S. (2014a). "Coping in Parents and Caregivers of Children with Autism Spectrum Disorders (ASD): a Review." *Review Journal of Autism and Developmental Disorders*, 1(3), 207–224. https://doi.org/10.1007/s40489-014-0021-x

[423] Barchel, D., Stolar, O., De-Haan, T., Ziv-Baran, T., Saban, N., Fuchs, D. O., Koren, G., & Berkovitch, M. (2019b). "Oral cannabidiol use in children with autism spectrum disorder to treat related symptoms and co-morbidities." *Frontiers in Pharmacology*, 9. https://doi.org/10.3389/fphar.2018.01521

[424] Ichtchenko, K., Hata, Y., Nguyen, T., Ullrich, B., Missler, M., Moomaw, C. R., & Südhof, T. C. (1995). "Neuroligin 1: A splice site-specific ligand for β-neurexins." *Cell*, 81(3), 435–443. https://doi.org/10.1016/0092-8674(95)90396-8

[425] Földy, C., Malenka, R. C., & Südhof, T. C. (2013). "Autism-Associated neuroligin-3 mutations commonly disrupt tonic endocannabinoid signaling." *Neuron*, 78(3), 498–509. https://doi.org/10.1016/j.neuron.2013.02.036

These observations reinforce the involvement of the ECS in the pathophysiology of autism.

Alzheimer's Disease

Alzheimer's disease (AD) is the most common neurodegenerative disease in the elderly and affects approximately 36 million people worldwide.[426] AD is characterized by progressive loss of recent memory and higher cognitive functions such as attention, judgment, and action planning, followed by disorientation and changes in behavior and mood.[427] These AD symptoms develop from brain tissue lesions spread across multiple brain regions, especially in the temporal, frontal, and parietal lobes, as well as the amygdala and cholinergic nuclei of the forebrain.[428,429,430]

Lesions in the cerebral cortex seen in AD are characterized by the accumulation of extracellular aggregates of amyloid beta-peptide (Aβ), which lead to the formation of amyloid plaques (also known as senile plaques) and intraneuronal neurofibrillary tangles, composed of filamentous aggregates of tau proteins.[431] The increased synthesis of Aβ peptide is related to the increased expression of an integral glycoprotein called amyloid precursor protein (APP), which occurs in the face of a punctual gene mutation (missense) on chromosome 21. In addition to the increased expression of APP, there are also alterations in the expression of presenilin-1 (PSEN1) and presenilin-2 (PSEN2), which result in changes in the proteolysis of APP by the gamma-secretase complex, leading to an increase in the ratio of Aβ42/40

---

[426] Prince M, Prina M, Guerchet M. "World Alzheimer Report 2013: Journey of caring: an analysis of long-term care for dementia." *London: Alzheimer's Disease International*; 2013. 92 p. http://www.alz.co.uk/research/WorldAlzheimerReport2013.pdf.

[427] Burns, A. (2009). "Alzheimer's disease: on the verges of treatment and prevention." *Lancet Neurology*, 8(1), 4–5. https://doi.org/10.1016/s1474-4422(08)70271-0

[428] Arendt, T. (2009). "Synaptic degeneration in Alzheimer's disease." *Acta Neuropathologica*, 118(1), 167–179. https://doi.org/10.1007/s00401-009-0536-x

[429] Braak, H., & Braak, E. (1991). "Neuropathological stageing of Alzheimer-related changes." *Acta Neuropathologica*, 82(4), 239–259. https://doi.org/10.1007/bf00308809

[430] Iulita, M. F., & Cuello, A. C. (2014). "Nerve growth factor metabolic dysfunction in Alzheimer's disease and Down syndrome." *Trends in Pharmacological Sciences*, 35(7), 338–348. https://doi.org/10.1016/j.tips.2014.04.010

[431] Glenner, G. G., & Wong, C. W. (1984). "Alzheimer's disease: Initial report of the purification and characterization of a novel cerebrovascular amyloid protein." *Biochemical and Biophysical Research Communications*, 120(3), 885–890. https://doi.org/10.1016/s0006-291x(84)80190-4

protein fragments in the brain.[432,433,434] This condition favors the formation and aggregation of Aβ42 oligomers that induce loss of synapses and neurotoxicity in AD.[435]

Another mechanism involved in the pathophysiology of AD refers to the nerve growth factor (NGF) pathway, of which levels are reduced due to the low expression of its precursor, pro-NGF, and the degradation of mature neurotrophins. This condition favors the reduction of endogenous trophic support to cholinergic neurons of the basal forebrain.[436] The reduction of NGF availability at the cortical level implies, among other conditions, the atrophy of the basal ganglia and, consequently, the reduction of cognitive functions.[437]

Low NGF production also leads to reduced activation of receptor tyrosine kinase A (TrkA), both in the basal forebrain and in the cerebral cortex, and causes imbalances in the levels of the p75NTR neurotrophin receptor. The imbalance of TrkA and p75NTR may favor the reduction of trophic responses in the brain and promote the activation of pro-apoptotic signaling pathways, such as the JNK protein kinase pathway (c-Jun N-terminal kinase), contributing to neurodegeneration.

In this context, Mufson et al.,[438] when studying hippocampus samples from patients with AD, observed low levels of NGF and hyperphosphorylation of JNK, findings that were correlated with the degree of cognitive impairment of patients. The degradation of mature neurotrophins further compromises

---

[432] De Strooper, B., Vassar, R., & Golde, T. E. (2010). "The secretases: enzymes with therapeutic potential in Alzheimer disease." *Nature Reviews Neurology*, 6(2), 99–107. https://doi.org/10.1038/nrneurol.2009.218

[433] Wolfe, M. S., Xia, W., Moore, C., Leatherwood, D. D., Ostaszewski, B. L., Rahmati, T., Donkor, I. O., & Selkoe, D. J. (1999). "Peptidomimetic probes and molecular modeling suggest that Alzheimer's Γ-Secretase is an Intramembrane-Cleaving aspartyl protease." *Biochemistry*, 38(15), 4720–4727. https://doi.org/10.1021/bi982562p

[434] Williamson, J., Goldman, J., & Marder, K. (2009). "Genetic aspects of Alzheimer disease." *The Neurologist*, 15(2), 80–86. https://doi.org/10.1097/nrl.0b013e318187e76b

[435] Supnet, C., & Bezprozvanny, I. (2010). "The dysregulation of intracellular calcium in Alzheimer disease." *Cell Calcium*, 47(2), 183–189. https://doi.org/10.1016/j.ceca.2009.12.014

[436] Cuello, A. C., & Bruno, M. A. (2007). "The Failure in NGF Maturation and its Increased Degradation as the Probable Cause for the Vulnerability of Cholinergic Neurons in Alzheimer's Disease." *Neurochemical Research*, 32(6), 1041–1045. https://doi.org/10.1007/s11064-006-9270-0

[437] Iulita, M. F., & Cuello, A. C. (2014). "Nerve growth factor metabolic dysfunction in Alzheimer's disease and Down syndrome." *Trends in Pharmacological Sciences*, 35(7), 338–348. https://doi.org/10.1016/j.tips.2014.04.010

[438] Mufson, E. J., Counts, S., Perez, S. E., & Ginsberg, S. D. (2008). "Cholinergic system during the progression of Alzheimer's disease: therapeutic implications." *Expert Review of Neurotherapeutics*, 8(11), 1703–1718. https://doi.org/10.1586/14737175.8.11.1703

the expression of brain-derived neurotrophic factor (BDNF). There is strong scientific evidence that the cerebral cortex and hippocampus of AD patients contain low levels of messenger RNA (mRNA) for BDNF, as well as its translated protein. Given the key role of BDNF in memory formation, learning, and synaptic plasticity, it is plausible to observe cognitive deficits in AD patients.[439]

Prior to memory loss, researchers observed behavioral changes and cognitive deficits due to the neurodegeneration present in AD and changes in the intracellular calcium (Ca2+) signaling pathway. This pathway impairment is due to deficits in the function of the endoplasmic reticulum (ER), which functions as an intracellular store of Ca2+. Ito et al.[440] observed that fibroblasts from patients in the risk group for the development of AD showed increased activation, mediated by Ca2+, of inositol-1,4,5-trisphosphate receptors (IP3Rs), favoring the release of Ca2+ from stores intracellular cells and, consequently, the increase in the intracellular concentration of Ca2+. Despite its function as a second messenger, Ca2+ is toxic to neurons in high concentrations, as it leads to the production of reactive oxygen species (ROS) and nitrogen species (RNS) and to apoptosis.[441] The accumulation of Aβ peptide and the consequent disturbance of intracellular Ca2+ homeostasis favor excessive activation of the N-methyl-D-aspartate (NMDA) glutamate receptor, leading to excitotoxicity and neuronal death.[442]

AD's pathogenesis is also strongly related to neuroinflammation and oxidative stress, as the accumulation of senile plaques leads to brain tissue toxicity and activation of microglia and astrocytes that surround amyloid

---

[439] Ferrer, I., MarÍN, C., Rey, M. J. B., Ribalta, T., Goutan, E., Blanco, R., Tolosa, E., & Martı, E. (1999). "BDNF and full-length and truncated TRKB expression in Alzheimer's disease. Implications in therapeutic strategies." *Journal of Neuropathology and Experimental Neurology, 58*(7), 729–739. https://doi.org/10.1097/00005072-199907000-00007

[440] Ito, E., Oka, K., Etcheberrigaray, R., Nelson, T., McPhie, D. L., Tofel-Grehl, B., Gibson, G. E., & Alkon, D. L. (1994). "Internal Ca2+ mobilization is altered in fibroblasts from patients with Alzheimer's disease." *Proceedings of the National Academy of Sciences of the United States of America, 91*(2), 534–538. https://doi.org/10.1073/pnas.91.2.534

[441] Supnet, C., & Bezprozvanny, I. (2010). "The dysregulation of intracellular calcium in Alzheimer's disease." *Cell Calcium, 47*(2), 183–189. https://doi.org/10.1016/j.ceca.2009.12.014

[442] Smith, M. A., Nunomura, A., Lee, H. G., Zhu, X., Moreira, P. I., Ávila, J., & Perry, G. (2005). "Chronological primacy of oxidative stress in Alzheimer's disease." *Neurobiology of Aging, 26*(5), 579–580. https://doi.org/10.1016/j.neurobiolaging.2004.09.021

plaques.[443] This process triggers a cascade of pro-inflammatory pathways, resulting in the release of substances such as cytokines, chemokines, ROS, and proteolytic enzymes, which lead to local inflammation, neuronal death, and, consequently, to the cognitive and behavioral deficits observed in AD.[444] Amidst the activation of the inflammatory response, mitochondrial dysfunction also occurs since the accumulation of Aβ peptide compromises cellular respiration and favors oxidative stress, leading to different molecule damage such as nucleic acids, proteins, lipids, and the ER.[445] The change in the lipid structure of cell membrane microdomains (the so-called lipid rafts) associated with inflammatory responses, altered production of trophic factors, neurotransmitters and neuromodulators and cytoplasmic proteolysis, autophagy and activation of the ubiquitin-proteasome pathway (UPS), favor the neurodegeneration.[446]

Phytocannabinoids and Alzheimer's Disease

Experimental studies point to the crucial role of the ECS in AD-related processes such as neuroinflammation, excitotoxicity, oxidative stress, and mitochondrial dysfunction.[447,448,449]

A study conducted by Eubanks et al.[450] concluded that THC was able to inhibit the enzyme acetylcholinesterase (AChE) and the aggregation of β-amyloid peptides induced by AChE. According to this same study, THC is considerably more effective in reducing Aβ deposition when compared to drugs like

---

[443] Ahmed, A. B., Znassi, N., Château, M., & Kajava, A. V. (2014). "A structure-based approach to predict predisposition to amyloidosis." *Alzheimer's & Dementia, 11*(6), 681–690. https://doi.org/10.1016/j.jalz.2014.06.007

[444] Eikelenboom, P., Veerhuis, R., Scheper, W., Rozemüller, A., Van Gool, W. A., & Hoozemans, J. J. M. (2006). "The significance of neuroinflammation in understanding Alzheimer's disease." *Journal of Neural Transmission, 113*(11), 1685–1695. https://doi.org/10.1007/s00702-006-0575-6

[445] Chen, J. X., & Yan, S. S. (2010). "Role of mitochondrial amyloid-B in Alzheimer's disease." *Journal of Alzheimer's Disease, 20*(s2), S569–S578. https://doi.org/10.3233/jad-2010-100357

[446] Aso, E., & Ferrer, I. (2014). "Cannabinoids for treatment of Alzheimer's disease: moving toward the clinic." *Frontiers in Pharmacology, 5*. https://doi.org/10.3389/fphar.2014.00037

[447] *Ibid*

[448] Maji, S. K., Schubert, D., Rivier, C., Lee, S., Rivier, J., & Riek, R. (2008). "Amyloid as a depot for the formulation of Long-Acting drugs." *PLOS Biology, 6*(2), e17. https://doi.org/10.1371/journal.pbio.0060017

[449] Watt, G., & Karl, T. (2017). "In vivo Evidence for Therapeutic Properties of Cannabidiol (CBD) for Alzheimer's Disease." *Frontiers in Pharmacology, 8*. https://doi.org/10.3389/fphar.2017.00020

[450] Eubanks, L. M., Rogers, C. J., Beuscher, A. E., Koob, G. F., Olson, A. J., Dickerson, T. J., & Janda, K. D. (2006). "A Molecular Link between the Active Component of Marijuana and Alzheimer's Disease Pathology." *Molecular Pharmaceutics, 3*(6), 773–777. https://doi.org/10.1021/mp060066m

donepezil and tacrine. In the *in vitro* study carried out by Currais et al.,[451] THC had a protective effect as it eliminated Aβ deposits and the production of induced eicosanoids in MC65 cells, thus attenuating the progressive inflammation present in AD. In another study, Iuvone et al.[452] showed the neuroprotective effect of cannabidiol (CBD) on Aβ-induced toxicity in PC12 cells. CBD treatment increased cell survival and decreased ROS production, lipid peroxidation, caspase-3 levels, DNA fragmentation, and intracellular calcium accumulation.

Cao et al.[453] tested the effects of THC on GSK-3β, showing efficacy in decreasing Aβ levels and GSK-3β phosphorylation in a dose-dependent manner at low concentrations in mouse neuroblastoma (N2A) cells. The Wnt signaling cascade and the action of CBD on PC12 cells were related in the study by Esposito et al.,[454] demonstrating the action of the cannabinoid in inhibiting tau protein hyperphosphorylation in Aβ previously stimulated *in vitro*, in which the inhibition of hyperphosphorylation leads to the formation of fibrillar tangles (NFTs), this effect being associated with the reduction of p-GSK3β, an active phosphorylated GSK-3β, resulting in the rescue of the Wnt/β-catenin pathway.

Behavioral changes are one of the main clinical manifestations observed in AD. A clinical study including 15 patients undergoing treatment with dronabinol (a synthetic analog of THC) showed a decline in the severity of behavioral changes in addition to weight gain in the analyzed patients.[455] In contrast, two pilot studies, including eight patients with AD, demonstrated a reduction in total hours of nocturnal agitation and behavioral disturbances

---

[451] Currais, A., Quehenberger, O., Armando, A. M., Daugherty, D. J., Maher, P., & Schubert, D. (2016). "Amyloid proteotoxicity initiates an inflammatory response blocked by cannabinoids." *Npj Aging and Mechanisms of Disease*, 2(1). https://doi.org/10.1038/npjamd.2016.12

[452] Iuvone, T., Esposito, G., Esposito, R., Santamaria, R., Di Rosa, M., & Izzo, A. A. (2004). "Neuroprotective effect of cannabidiol, a non-psychoactive component from Cannabis sativa, on beta-amyloid-induced toxicity in PC12 cells." *Journal of Neurochemistry*, 89(1), 134–141. https://doi.org/10.1111/j.1471-4159.2003.02327.x

[453] Cao, C., Li, Y., Liu, H., Bai, G., Mayl, J., Lin, X., Sutherland, K., Nabar, N. R., & Cai, J. (2014). "The potential therapeutic effects of THC on Alzheimer's disease." *Journal of Alzheimer's Disease*, 42(3), 973–984. https://doi.org/10.3233/jad-140093

[454] Esposito, G., De Filippis, D., Carnuccio, R., Izzo, A. A., & Iuvone, T. (2005). "The marijuana component cannabidiol inhibits β-amyloid-induced tau protein hyperphosphorylation through Wnt/β-catenin pathway rescue in PC12 cells." *Journal of Molecular Medicine*, 84(3), 253–258. https://doi.org/10.1007/s00109-005-0025-1

[455] Volicer, Ladislav, Marilyn Stelly, Judith Morris, Joseph McLaughlin, and Beverly J. Volicer. "Effects of Dronabinol on Anorexia and Disturbed Behavior in Patients with Alzheimer's Disease." *International Journal of Geriatric Psychiatry 12*, no. 9 (1997): 913-919. Accessed October 25, 2023. https://doi.org/10.1002/(SICI)1099-1166(199709)12:9<913::AID-GPS663>3.0.CO;2-D.

during a period of dronabinol treatment.[456,457] In addition, the use of nabilone (another synthetic THC with alterations in the chemical structure) proved to be effective in reducing aggressiveness in patients with advanced-stage AD who were using anxiolytic and antipsychotic drugs.[458] Nabilone mimics THC but is more potent than other analogs, acting on both CB_1 and CB_2 receptors.[459]

A literature review conducted by Liu et al.[460] pointed out that synthetic cannabinoids analogous to THC (nabilone and dronabinol) may offer less risk and more efficacy than antipsychotic medications when used in patients with AD. A clinical trial that sought to evaluate the efficacy and safety of nabilone for reducing agitation associated with AD showed that treatment with this drug can be effective in reducing agitation; however, side effects such as sedation and cognitive impairment were equally significant.[461] A meta-analysis reviewing six clinical trials on the subject showed that there is a trend towards reduced agitation after treatment with nabilone, and sedation was the main adverse event reported. The study authors concluded that the treatment has a potential benefit and that further trials may help to better understand the effects of this drug.[462] Perhaps the use of THC associated with other cannabinoids can minimize the adverse events indicated by previous studies.

In a double-blind randomized controlled trial (RTC), Ruthirakuhan et al.[463] demonstrated the beneficial effects of nabilone in patients with moderate to

---

[456] Walther, S., Mahlberg, R., Eichmann, U., & Kunz, D. (2006). "Delta-9-tetrahydrocannabinol for nighttime agitation in severe dementia." *Psychopharmacology, 185*(4), 524–528. https://doi.org/10.1007/s00213-006-0343-1

[457] Walther, S., & Halpern, M. T. (2010). Cannabinoids and Dementia: A review of clinical and preclinical data. *Pharmaceuticals, 3*(8), 2689–2708. https://doi.org/10.3390/ph3082689

[458] Passmore, M. J. (2007). "The cannabinoid receptor agonist nabilone for the treatment of dementia-related agitation." *International Journal of Geriatric Psychiatry, 23*(1), 116–117. https://doi.org/10.1002/gps.1828

[459] Lemberger, L., & Rowe, H. (1975). "Clinical pharmacology of nabilone, a cannabinol derivative." *Clinical Pharmacology & Therapeutics, 18*(6), 720–726. https://doi.org/10.1002/cpt1975186720

[460] Liu, C. S., Chau, S., Ruthirakuhan, M., Lanctôt, K. L., & Herrmann, N. (2015). "Cannabinoids for the treatment of agitation and aggression in Alzheimer's disease." *CNS Drugs, 29*(8), 615–623. https://doi.org/10.1007/s40263-015-0270-y

[461] Herrmann, N., Ruthirakuhan, M., Gallagher, D., Verhoeff, N. P. L., Kiss, A., Black, S. E., & Lanctôt, K. L. (2019). "Randomized Placebo-Controlled Trial of Nabilone for agitation in Alzheimer's Disease." *American Journal of Geriatric Psychiatry, 27*(11), 1161–1173. https://doi.org/10.1016/j.jagp.2019.05.002

[462] Ruthirakuhan, M., Lanctôt, K. L., Vieira, D. S. R., & Herrmann, N. (2019). "Natural and synthetic cannabinoids for agitation and aggression in Alzheimer's disease." *The Journal of Clinical Psychiatry, 80*(2). https://doi.org/10.4088/jcp.18r12617

[463] Ruthirakuhan, M., Herrmann, N., Gallagher, D., Andreazza, A. C., Kiss, A., Verhoeff, N. P. L., Black, S. E., & Lanctôt, K. L. (2019). "Investigating the safety and efficacy of nabilone for the treatment of agitation in

severe stage AD. The authors compared the effects of using nabilone (0.5-2 mg) to placebo treatment for six weeks and observed nabilone's positive effects on agitation, pain, and weight loss in patients with AD, with beneficial consequences on these patients' quality of life, including improving the well-being of caregivers and lower expenses with hospitalizations and other health care services in general.

Given these findings, the search for therapeutic alternatives seems to potentially target several signaling pathways, such as the one responsible for regulating Wnt/β-catenin and tau protein hyperphosphorylation, leading to a reduction in symptoms such as aggressiveness and mood disorders.

---

patients with moderate-to-severe Alzheimer's disease: Study protocol for a cross-over randomized controlled trial." *Contemporary Clinical Trials Communications, 15*, 100385. https://doi.org/10.1016/j.conctc.2019.100385

Dr. Bearman's Clinical Standards

How extensive should a physician visit be when recommending cannabis or other nonprescription, alternative, complementary therapies? Unfortunately, the answer is subject to the whims of regional medical boards and whether the board views a doctor as a primary care physician or a cannabinoid medicine specialist.

As the former medical director and director of the Health Services Department of the Santa Barbara Regional Health Authority (SBRHA, now known as CenCal Health), it is the opinion of the author that in many cases, the recommending physician is not acting as the primary care physician but as a specialist in much the same way as a physician operating within a methadone maintenance clinic setting.

The problem is that it needs to be more objective regarding what standards are appropriate for an alternative or complementary medical treatment and what the medical board requires. Since this is open to interpretation, physicians recommending cannabis need to practice and document more on the conservative side. The author served for 14 years as medical director of SBRHA/CenCal and stated that there is a wide variability of medical practice standards, subjective application, and nature of such standards.

There are several practice standards currently being used. It appears that some US states and local regions apply these standards with great vigor when recommending cannabis for medicinal use. These standards are based on Dr. Bearman's over two decades of recommending medical cannabis in California, the first place in the world that explicitly re-legalized its medical use after the UN Single Convention on Narcotic Drugs in 1961. These standards shape the recommending doctor's interaction with patients.

Patient Evaluation

A documented in-person medical evaluation and collection of relevant clinical history should include the patient's history of present illness, past medical and surgical history, alcohol and other substance use history, physical exam, plus the diagnosis that requires the cannabis recommendation.

Physician-Patient Relationship

The Association of Medical Boards recommends the following regarding guidelines: Physicians must have documented that an appropriate physician-patient relationship has been established prior to providing a recommendation, attestation, or authorization for marijuana to the patient. *The Medical Board of California (MBC)* guidelines include the following for recommending cannabis:

- A verified doctor-patient relationship
- Good faith history and physical
- Review records
- Create a plan with objectives
- Diagnosis that will benefit from the use of cannabis

The author takes issue with having a plan with objectives because it is not information required by the California State Health Department for Medicaid-managed care programs.

Vital Signs

The medical exam should include recording the patient's vital signs. Doctors recommending cannabis should take pulse, weight, and blood pressure.

Dr. Bearman's Practice Pattern as a Reference Guide

Doctors have different standards that they hold themselves to. Sometimes, with cannabis medicine, for medico-legal reasons, doctors may want to practice defensive medicine. This includes pre-visit screening, getting the patient's relevant old medical records, written and oral history, and providing the patient a brief overview of medicinal cannabis, including a discussion of side effects and routes of administration. Doctors should also cover dosage, THC, CBD, terpenes, and Marinol. Doctors may also wish to explore the option of not utilizing cannabis-based medicine and possibly other alternative treatments. This is a very prudent way to make recommendations to a new patient, and it helps to build a doctor-patient relationship.

The best advice in practicing cannabinoid medicine is to treat cannabis and cannabinoids as any other therapeutic agent.

1. **Pre-visit screening:** Doctors may wish to screen all potential new cannabinoid medicine patients on the phone and ask them for their diagnosis and what documentation they have, the treatment they have received, and the last time they sought medical attention for the condition they are seeking the cannabis recommendation for.
2. **Have educational material in the waiting room:** Have educational materials assembled to give the patient that explain the mechanisms of action, the endocannabinoid system, cannabis, cannabinoids, and terpenes.
3. **Appointment length:** The first appointment should take between 25 and 60 minutes, depending upon the complexity of the case.
4. **History:** Doctors might require patients to bring both old records and complete a multi-page history form. The author also takes an oral history from the patient at the time of the visit.
5. **Physical exam:** Perform a reasonable general physical, including vital signs, with a particular examination of the body part or organ system principally involved in the patient's medical condition being considered for cannabis recommendation.
6. **Follow-up and referral as medically appropriate:** Make appropriate referrals when indicated. As a matter of continuity of care, send consultation reports, progress notes, and care plans to specialists who are actively involved in the patient's care management.
7. **Practice good medicine:** Doctors who practice good medicine have little to worry about when recommending cannabis. Chances are that patients will not have a problem with law enforcement. Still, on some occasions, doctors may need to testify in support of their patients in court. Don't dwell on that as a possible big drain on professional time. The necessity for going to court to explain medicinal cannabis is becoming rarer, and the time is billable. It is also par for the course as a doctor choosing to utilize cannabis in their patient's treatment.
8. **Record keeping:** Keep good records. This is the best protection against an over-zealous medical board. Do adequate documentation. History-taking and chart documentation need to be done with the possibility of needing to rely on detailed documentation records in court. There is often a distinction between chart notes required or expected of a specialist and those of a primary care provider. The consultant often focuses mainly on the specific specialist issues before them. In this context, what is primarily determined is whether the patient has a condition that could benefit from the use of

cannabis. There needs to be sufficient documentation to justify making such a recommendation.

Educational Discussion

There are many misconceptions about cannabis. Both patients and physicians alike have grown up having been presented with misinformation and falsehoods regarding cannabis and likely never learned about cannabinoids and the endocannabinoid system. It can help the patient feel at ease by framing medicinal cannabis by history, modern clinical use, and science. Those who have experience using cannabis recreationally may think they understand the medical applications.

The following topics are typically covered in the initial discussion:

- The voluntary medical cannabis identification state card
- The science of ECS and cannabis
- The dose and route of administration
- The common side effects
- Explain the mechanism of action of retrograde inhibition

Data Needed to Document Justification for Recommendation

How much data a physician needs to know to and/or begin to surmise and eventually conclude that a patient would benefit from the use of cannabis for medical purposes varies, but the information required is relatively straightforward. This information includes:

- The patient diagnosis and/or medical condition
- A medical history

Part IV: The Future

The discovery and research elucidating the endocannabinoid system is dramatically re-shaping healthcare through the incorporation of cannabis and cannabinoids into clinical practice. This book concludes with a look forward from the perspective of the authors' and the scientist who started it all, Dr. Raphael Mechoulam.

The Future of Cannabis Medicine

As described in previous chapters, much is already known about cannabis's mechanisms of action in humans. What is known is exciting and promising in the treatment of many serious illnesses. Unfortunately, cannabis's Schedule I status in the United States and similar prohibitions worldwide have prevented the actual human clinical trials required for its proper integration into healthcare.

One of the most significant impacts on the field of cannabinoid medicine is cannabis being labeled as a Schedule I drug under the Controlled Substances Act of 1971. Removing cannabis from the schedule system in the Controlled Substances Act is starting to look like a strong possibility. As of this writing, there are multiple (many bipartisan) pieces of legislation—that include the aforementioned policy change—filed or passed through the House of Representatives and various subcommittees. Beyond the United States, cannabis policies are changing worldwide and will continue to change.

With the legalization of **"adult use"** cannabis, or the non-medicinal use by people over 21, there must be more education for all healthcare professionals. Whether or not a patient is diagnosed with a severe or chronic illness, where cannabis is legal, it will be incorporated as a common herb. Past and potential policy changes have altered existing approaches to the medicinal use of cannabis and will continue to shift as legalization spreads. Physicians, nurses, and all other healthcare professionals must be able to have honest and well-informed discussions with the patients they serve about the endocannabinoid system, the practice of cannabinoid medicine, and cannabis use for any reason.

More education for healthcare professionals is the most critical thing that can and should happen in the future to compensate for the snail's pace of research. It has been almost 60 years since Dr. Mechoulam first isolated and identified CBD and THC. Until he passed away in 2023, Dr. Mechoulam remained at the forefront of the research. Our work with him in producing the foreword to this book and some of his final observations guided this chapter, which lists what the authors believe is the future of cannabinoid medicine.

Personalized Medicine

More research will reveal how plant synergies work in different patients, paving the way for personalized medicinal uses of cannabis. Dr. Mechoulam was optimistic that the future holds more personalized medicine. In the interview with *Cannabis Now Magazine*, he stated:

> *I expect that by proper supervision, we shall have "personalized medicine," as obviously different cannabinoids may be needed for different conditions. This is of high importance as physicians at present are reluctant to prescribe just "cannabis" without exact knowledge of the levels of THC and CBD and published detailed scientific-medical data on the use of cannabis in specific diseases. I believe that bringing cannabis as a medicine to parallel the use of approved drugs will be a major step forward.*

Better Analysis & Standardization

There continues to be a need for standardization with cannabis and other herbal medicinal products. All cannabis products should be lab tested, and display the product contents and dosage on the label.

All cannabis regulations require testing for cannabinoids, pesticides, and toxins. Unfortunately, testing labs do not operate by a common set of standards. Reports of lab shopping for favorable tests in many states have become a growing concern. As labs become more consistent in analysis, cannabis products will also become more standardized, which is necessary for proper research, dosing, and recommending or prescribing full-spectrum cannabis and cannabis medicines. In turn, better analysis and standardization will facilitate more significant research on both the individual constituents of cannabis and the synergies they create.

Better Understanding of Both Individual Cannabinoids & Phytochemical Synergies

Once legislation changes how cannabis is treated, there will undoubtedly be more research on all cannabinoids, including CBD, THC, CBG, varin cannabinoids (like THCV and CBDV), acid cannabinoids (like THCa, CBDa, and CBGa), and many that are today yet to be identified. There will also be more research on other notable individual constituents found in cannabis, such as terpenes and flavonoids, particularly the flavonoids that are mostly unique to cannabis: the cannflavins.

While the focus may be on these individual compounds, there must also be robust research on full spectrum synergies or how the array of phytocompounds work together to create or induce the specific effects of different cannabis varieties and preparations.

More Professionalism

With better education of healthcare professionals, there will also be improved professional standards in the healthcare industry. There is a need for pharmacists, physicians, nurses, therapists, and caregivers to understand the endocannabinoid system and operate by professional standards surrounding cannabis and cannabinoid medicines. The Society of Cannabis Clinicians (SCC) and the American Academy of Cannabinoid Medicine (AACM) have created standards for physicians. The future will show greater adoption and unity in the healthcare profession behind such standardization.

Cannabis dispensaries, which act as pharmacies for many patients, will also be expected to staff better-trained professionals who operate by common standards preventing salespeople from dispensing medical advice. Medical advice should be dispensed at pharmacies by prescription so a pharmacist can make sure patients receive proper guidance to use the safest and most effective products possible.

Increased Use of Cannabinoids in All Forms

Current trends are evident: more people will use cannabinoids. This usage includes the increased use of off-label synthetic Δ^9-THC, Marinol (dronabinol), increased use of pharmaceutical cannabis tincture products Epidiolex (cannabidiol) and Sativex (nabiximols), increased use of botanical preparations of cannabis, as well as increased non-medical use by adults. With changing laws and greater acceptance of the general safety of cannabis, there will, in turn, be an increase in home cultivation and DIY remedies.

More Research & Better Clinical Trials

Currently, in the United States, Schedule I status prevents human clinical trials from taking place. The vast majority of cannabis research thus far has been done in lab settings using human cells and isolated cannabinoids. While this preclinical research is valuable and certainly can inform medical practice and future research, actual clinical trials conducted with humans are required. This need will continue to grow, and ultimately, there will be a boom in clinical cannabis and cannabinoid studies in the future.

As Dr. Mechoulam stated in an interview with Cannabis Now Magazine[464] in 2015:

> Clinical research with cannabinoids is difficult to undertake in any country. In Israel, cannabinoid research has been done in all universities, but financial support is limited, as in all fields ...Clinical research, as in all developed countries, requires approvals by hospital and government committees, which demand strict supervision.

Some clinical trials have been conducted in Israel and inform the practice of cannabinoid medicine today. Researchers everywhere will and should one day have the ability and funding to conduct clinical trials better to understand all elements of cannabis and its therapeutic properties so that education and knowledge are allowed to advance.

The most significant barrier to research and acceptance into mainstream medicine is that cannabis is Schedule I. Moving cannabis to Schedule III, as was recommended by the Department of Health and Human Services in 2023, would make research much more attainable. However, many activists support de-scheduling cannabis and treating it like the plant it is, which is more in line with the historical role of plant medicine. Most Congressional legalization proposals in the United States now include the complete removal of cannabis from the Controlled Substances Act. Both a re-scheduling and a de-scheduling would significantly reduce the barriers to research and provide a path for the most critical studies, including more studies on military veterans with PTSD, cancer, and autoimmune disorders, and more honest studies about potential harms.

Military Veterans with Post-Traumatic Stress Disorder

US military veterans suffering from the mental trauma of war widely use cannabis, and usage has increased since the Vietnam War. Current pharmaceutical treatments are inadequate, and for military veterans from Iraq and Afghanistan in particular, their treatment or lack thereof often results in tragedy. More veterans under 40 die by suicide than any other age

---

[464] Daw, Jeremy. (2018, May 9). "Dr. Mechoulam talks about the future of Cannabis Research." *Cannabis Now*. Retrieved April 10, 2022, from https://cannabisnow.com/dr-mechoulam-talks-the-future-of-cannabis-research/

group. According to the Department of Veterans Affairs (VA), in 2019, over 7,000 veterans took their own lives.[465]

In 2009, Dr. Sue Sisley initiated the crucial work of undergoing a clinical trial to understand the effects of cannabis treatment for this specific high-risk population. Such trials are necessary to provide veterans with the best care possible and prevent suicides. Dr. Sisely finally concluded her clinical trial after over ten years of navigating bureaucracy to use botanical cannabis in her study intended for the treatment of US military veterans in Colorado and Arizona. Despite overcoming numerous roadblocks, such as receiving moldy cannabis from the government to work with, her trial concluded that further research was warranted.[466] Unfortunately, she says her study ultimately couldn't overcome many of these roadblocks, notably that many veterans in her patient sample returned the low-quality government-grown cannabis that was prescribed.

More Studies on Cancer

A growing number of cancer patients are turning to cannabis to either treat their symptoms or attempt to shrink their tumors. While there is a growing and promising body of research surrounding cannabis and cancer, the future holds actual clinical trials, studies into different types of cancers, and the ability to customize cannabis medicines to treat specific tumors in specific patients. Dr. Joe Goldstrich does an excellent job laying out the current body of research and the areas of future study in *The Cannabis-Cancer Connection* (2023).

More Studies on Autoimmune Disease and Disorders

Some of the most widespread medicinal uses of cannabis, with or without the guidance of a doctor, is the treatment of the symptoms of autoimmune diseases and disorders such as epilepsy, multiple sclerosis, Crohn's disease and IBD, fibromyalgia, rheumatoid arthritis, psoriasis, and more. Cannabis use in these patient populations would benefit from clinical trials and more significant research.

---

[465] United States Department of Veteran Affairs. (2019). *2019 National Veteran Suicide Prevention Annual Report.* Retrieved April 11, 2022, from https://www.mentalhealth.va.gov/docs/data-sheets/2019/2019_National_Veteran_Suicide_Prevention_Annual_Report_508.pdf

[466] Abbott, D. (2021, July 8). "Pot and PTSD: Study shines light on need to end cannabis prohibition as researchers seek alternatives for lousy research weedk alternatives for Lousy Research Weed." *Tucson Weekly.* Retrieved April 11, 2022, from https://www.tucsonweekly.com/tucson/pot-and-ptsd-study-shines-light-on-need-to-end-cannabis-prohibition-as-researchers-seek-alternatives-for-lousy-research-weed/Content?oid=30972767

In an interview with Yubal Zolotov of Fundación Canna, Dr. Mechoulam stated:

> *I expect that once we acquire more knowledge, we can treat more patients with different kinds of medical conditions, greater numbers than today. For instance, there are 80 autoimmune diseases in which the body attacks itself. Based on studies in the lab, mine, and others, it is plausible that cannabidiol (CBD) can treat at least some of them. So there is lots to do.*[467]

More Studies on ADD/ADHD, Anxiety, and Other Mental Conditions

There is a range of mental conditions, such as ADD, ADHD, depression, and anxiety, for which cannabis provides symptom relief. The future holds thorough clinical trials to understand better how different chemical profiles produced by cannabis affect the symptoms of these conditions and how to guide the treatment of these patients.

Honest Study About Potential Harms

When medical students become doctors, they take an oath to "first, do no harm." The vast majority of cannabis users, regardless of whether they have a diagnosed medical condition, will have no serious side effects from cannabis because it is very safe. But where there is a contraindication and potential for harm in specific populations, particularly those already predisposed to psychotic disorders, we must have more rigorous and serious studies to understand why and prevent adverse outcomes. In a Fundación Canna interview, Dr. Mechoulam stated:

> *This is a much more controversial topic. Based on some evidence, it may help several mental conditions, such as schizophrenia. Currently, post-traumatic stress is the only mental indication that is eligible for medical cannabis, according to Israeli regulations. We did a small study with human subjects, which had very good results. But the government is very careful about approving new mental indications.*

---

[467] Zolotov Yuval (Tuby) "Meet the experts: Interview with professor Raphael Mechoulam." *Fundación CANNA: Scientific studies and cannabis testing.* Retrieved April 10, 2022, from https://www.fundacion-canna.es/en/meet-experts-interview-professor-raphael-mechoulam

This field of study remains controversial, challenging, and guided by politics more than science. Hence, the concern about a lack of honest studies surrounding cannabis and mental health is not unfounded. Psychiatrist and researcher Zerrin Atakan wrote in a study in *Therapeutic Advances in Psychopharmacology*[468]:

> *What makes someone more susceptible to its negative effects is not yet known; however, there are some emerging vulnerability factors, ranging from certain genes to personality characteristics.*

Thorough clinical trials can better identify vulnerable populations and prevent adverse outcomes.

Policy Change

The future undoubtedly holds more changes in cannabis policy worldwide, particularly concerning research and education. Dr. Mechoulam was optimistic about the future of therapeutic cannabis use, concluding in his remarks to Fundación CANNA:

> *The medical potential of cannabis is huge, and we should not miss out. I believe that this potential is no longer being ignored, and that's why I'm satisfied with the recent developments of medical cannabis policies. I think that in the future, more and more patients will have access to medical products based on cannabis and cannabinoids. Science will continue to accumulate data, and we will know more. While the use of medical cannabis is undoubtedly going to expand, my hope is that it will do so in a rational way.*

---

[468] Atakan, Z. (2012, December). "Cannabis, a complex plant: Different compounds and different effects on individuals." *Therapeutic advances in psychopharmacology.* Retrieved April 10, 2022, from https://www.ncbi.nlm.nih.gov/pmc/articles/PMC3736954/

Glossary

Adenosine Triphosphate (ATP)
Adenosine triphosphate (ATP) is the energy source for use and storage at the cellular level.[469]

Adipose Tissue
Adipose tissue is also referred to as "fatty tissue" or body fat and refers to connective tissue mainly composed of fat cells called adipocytes.

Adult Use
The term "adult use" refers to the non-medicinal use of cannabis.

Allopathic Medical Approach
The allopathic medical approach is the mainstream approach used by Western medical practitioners. The allopathic medical approach is to treat symptoms and diseases with drugs, radiation, or surgery. *See also Integrative Medical Approach.*

Analgesia
Analgesia is the absence of pain.

Anandamide
N-arachidonoyl ethanolamide (AEA), referred to as anandamide, is one of the best-known endogenous cannabinoids and acts as an endogenous agonist of CB1 and CB2 receptors, much like THC. Anandamide is nicknamed "the bliss molecule." Ananda is a Sanskrit word that translates roughly as "bliss" and is thought to contribute to "the runner's high" experienced after vigorous exercise. *See also Endogenous Cannabinoids.*

---

[469] Dunn J, Grider MH. Physiology, Adenosine Triphosphate. [Updated 2023 Feb 13]. In: StatPearls [Internet]. Treasure Island (FL): StatPearls Publishing; 2024 Jan-. Available from: https://www.ncbi.nlm.nih.gov/books/NBK553175/

Anxiolytic
A drug that reduces anxiety.

Apoptosis
Cannabinoids can create a positive feedback loop, increasing stress to the point where the cancer cell self-destructs. This self-destruction is called "apoptosis."

Bioavailability
The proportion of a drug or other substance that enters the bloodstream and is able to have an active effect.[470]

Bud
Bud *see Flower.*

Cannabinoid
Cannabinoids are chemical compounds created both by plants (phytocannabinoids) and animal bodies (endogenous cannabinoids) that regulate the endocannabinoid systems of animals. *See also Endocannabinoid System.*

Cannabis
The term "cannabis" refers to all plants in the *Cannabis* genus, including industrial hemp and plants grown for their resinous, therapeutic flowers. The definitions have evolved. Cannabis flowers are known legally and in widespread use in the United States as "marijuana," a term deliberately chosen to create a negative racist association with users of the plant in Northern Mexico, who coined the slang term. Today, the term "cannabis" is used to replace "marijuana" in most instances, but it also refers to hemp plants grown for flowers and industrial uses. *See also Hemp.*

Combustion
Combustion refers to smoking cannabis because it requires the burning, and therefore combustion, of plant material to create smoke that is inhaled.

---

[470] Oxford English Dictionary

Cultivar

Cultivar means "cultivated variety" and is meant to distinguish the finished flowers of the cannabis plant as a unique product of not just the plant's genetics but also the environmental conditions provided by the farmer. *See also Strain* and *Variety*.

Dabbing

Dabbing is a form of vaporization that uses a torch to heat a glass, ceramic, or titanium element to vaporize a small amount (or "dab") of cannabis concentrate for inhalation.

Decarboxylation

Decarboxylation is the process of an acidic cannabinoid converting to its active form through the loss of a carboxyl group to its molecular structure and requires heat and time.

Dysphoria

Dysphoria is excessive, unpleasant euphoria, or "cannabis high.".

Endogenous Cannabinoids

Endogenous cannabinoids, or endocannabinoids, are produced within animal bodies and bind with endocannabinoid receptors.

Endocannabinoid System (ECS)

The ECS is a group of receptors comprising a complex regulatory system throughout the human brain, body, and central and peripheral nervous systems. The ECS creates and maintains the body's internal stability (homeostasis) by adjusting the flow of neurotransmitters and regulating bodily functions, including appetite, sleep, emotion, and movement.[471]

Entheogen

Entheogens are substances, usually herbs, that enhance spiritual connection.

---

[471] Colorado State University. (2018, June 1). *The Endocannabinoid System, Our Universal Regulator*. Journal of Young Investigators. Retrieved January 31, 2022, from https://www.jyi.org/2018-june/2018/6/1/the-endocannabinoid-system-our-universal-regulator1

Entourage Effect
Entourage effect is a theory that all of the therapeutic constituents of cannabis act together to create their effects,[472] that is, the combination of all the compounds present in the plant is more effective than its isolated elements. The entourage effect is not unique to cannabis but can be applied to all herbal medicines.

Euphoriphobia
Euphoriphobia is the fear of feeling "high" from cannabis use.

Flavonoids
Flavonoids are plant pigments responsible for the colors of plants, including cannabis, that also have medicinal properties.

Flowers
The term "flowers" refers to the flowering inflorescences of the female cannabis plant. Also colloquially referred to as "buds" or "nugs," these resinous flowers contain the most usable medicine.

Full Extract Cannabis Oil (FECO)
When made correctly, FECO is a highly-concentrated cannabis oil that includes as much of the full spectrum of compounds found in botanical cannabis as possible. FECO is an herbal product that is easy to make at home and sometimes available commercially. It is not a standardized, consistent product and can be made with various solvents and cannabis chemovars. FECO is sometimes referred to as Rick Simpson Oil (RSO) after the Canadian cancer patient who popularized its use online. RSO was initially made using naphtha (a toxic paint thinner). In contrast, FECO is made at home with food-grade alcohol or produced commercially using butane or carbon dioxide in licensed facilities. All commercially produced FECO must be laboratory-tested for potency, residual solvents, and toxins.

Free Radicals *see Reactive Oxygen Species.*

---

[472] Ben-Shabat, S., Fride, E., Sheskin, T., Tamiri, T., Rhee, M. H., Vogel, Z., Bisogno, T., De Petrocellis, L., Di Marzo, V., & Mechoulam, R. (1998). "An entourage effect: inactive endogenous fatty acid glycerol esters enhance 2-arachidonoyl-glycerol cannabinoid activity." *European Journal of Pharmacology, 353*(1), 23–31. https://doi.org/10.1016/s0014-2999(98)00392-6

Full Spectrum
The term full spectrum is used to describe cannabis-based medicines that utilize as much or all of the natural therapeutic molecules that the plant has to offer.

Hemp
The definition of "hemp" has evolved over time. All plants referred to as "hemp" belong to the *Cannabis* genus. Traditionally, hemp plants were varieties bred for their fiber and seeds, used to produce foods, paper, fabrics, and oils for bioplastics. Due to prohibition-inspired legal definitions, today, the term also refers to plants bred for resinous flowers that produce less than 0.3% Δ^9-THC.

Herbal Medicine
Herbal medicine refers to the medicinal use of foods, plants, fungi, and other natural botanical products that can have a therapeutic effect. *See also Nutraceutical.*

Homeostasis
Homeostasis is the state of internal balance, physical and chemical, of physiological systems' maintenance.

Hyperemesis
Hyperemesis is a medical condition characterized by excessive and severe bouts of vomiting.

Indica
Indica refers to varieties of cannabis that originated in the Hindu-Kush region at middle latitudes and high altitudes. They tend to be shorter, denser, darker, wider-leafed, and produce more resinous flowers. Most commercially available cannabis has been bred beyond this distinction, but the term also colloquially refers to varieties of cannabis that produce more relaxed and pain-relieving effects.

Integrative Medical Approach
Integrative care is a comprehensive treatment model that considers the human body as an indivisible entity. Integrative medical approaches seek to use nutrition, mental health, and exercise to prevent or lessen the need for allopathic medical interventions. *See also Allopathic Medical Approach.*

Marijuana *see Cannabis.*

Nutraceutical
Nutraceutical refers to foods and herbs that can impart a therapeutic benefit. *See also Herbal Medicine.*

Pathophysiology
Pathophysiology refers to the study of abnormal or disordered changes in body functions associated with disease processes.

Phytocannabinoids
Phytocannabinoids are cannabinoids produced by plants. *See also Cannabinoids.*

Psychoactive
Psychoactive refers to substances that cross the blood-brain barrier and actively affect the brain and perception. The term is often misused to refer to the psychotropic effects of cannabis and cannabinoids. *See also Psychotropic.*

Psychotropic
Psychotropic refers to substances that produce a "high," such as high-THC cannabis.

Pyrolysis
Pyrolysis refers to heating organic materials and initiating degradation. The term is used to refer to smoking cannabis.

Reactive Oxygen Species (ROS)
ROS is a type of unstable molecule that contains oxygen and easily reacts with other molecules in a cell. A build-up of reactive oxygen species in cells may cause damage to DNA, RNA, and proteins and may cause cell death. Reactive oxygen species are free radicals and are also referred to as "oxygen radicals" and "free radicals."[473]

---

[473]*NCI Dictionary of Cancer terms.* National Cancer Institute. (n.d.). Retrieved January 20, 2022, from https://www.cancer.gov/publications/dictionaries/cancer-terms/def/reactive-oxygen-species

Rick Simpson Oil (RSO)
Rick Simpson Oil (RSO) *See Full Extract Cannabis Oil (FECO).*

Ruderalis
Ruderalis varieties of cannabis evolved at higher latitudes in Russia in rocky terrains. They are short, fast finishing, and have the auto-flowering trait.

Sativa
Sativa refers to varieties of cannabis that originated on the equator. They tend to be taller, less dense, more brightly colored, have longer thin leaves, and take longer to finish. Most commercially available cannabis has been bred beyond this distinction, but the term also colloquially refers to varieties of cannabis that produce more stimulating and creativity-inducing effects.

Strain
Although the term "strain" has been commonly used to refer to varieties and cultivars of the cannabis plant, it is inaccurate because it refers to bacteria and viruses rather than plant varieties. The more appropriate terms are "variety" or "cultivar."

Substance Dependency
Substance dependency is defined as using a substance in such a manner that the consumption of that substance interferes with important aspects of a person's life, be it financial, occupational, educational, recreational, social, familial, or other important parts of life.

Suppositories
Suppositories are cannabis-infused medical preparation inserted into the vagina or rectum and absorbed internally.

Terpenes
Terpenes are aroma molecules found on most plants, including cannabis, that also have medicinal properties.

Titration
Titration means starting with a tiny dose and incrementally working it higher.

Trichome
Trichomes are resinous glands that grow on cannabis and contain the highest concentration of cannabinoids and terpenes.

Vaporization
Vaporization is the process of heating the volatile oils found in cannabis or other substances to convert them to inhalable gasses.

Variety
Variety or varietal refers to families of cannabis plants distinguished by their unique genetics, both those found growing in the wild and those resulting from a dedicated breeding program. This word is a more accurate replacement for "strain." *See also Cultivar* and *Strain.*

Index

11-hydroxy-THC, 54, 61, 68, 69, 82, 93
2-AG, 19, 20, 25, 119
Abrams, Donald, 60, 80
Acetylcholinesterase inhibitor, 46
Acupuncture, 9, 106, 109
ADD, 57, 73, 87, 156
Adenosine triphosphate, 27, 29, 31
ADHD, 26, 32, 57, 100, 101, 156
Adipogenesis, 22
Adipose tissue, 69, 82, 96
AEA, 19, 20, 25, 119, 136, 158
AIDS, 9, 80, 103
Albumin, 35
Alzheimer's disease, 40, 102, 131, 139, 140, 141, 142, 143, 144, 145
American Academy of Cannabinoid Medicine, 111, 153
American Medical Association, 14, 17
American Psychiatric Association, 89, 90, 91, 133
American Public Health Association, 17
American Society of Addiction Medicine, 115
Amino acids, 27, 48
Analgesia, 21, 31, 57, 82, 111
Analgesic, 13, 16, 31, 39, 40, 45, 47, 48, 55, 67, 71, 104, 110, 111, 113
Anandamide, 19, 20, 83, 110, 111, 136, 158
Anorexia, 102, 143
Anslinger, 17, 18
Antidepressant, 46, 135
Antiemetic, 41, 104, 128, 130
Antiepileptic drugs, 59, 71, 136
Anti-inflammatory, 29, 31, 38, 39, 40, 41, 44, 45, 47, 48, 57, 67, 78, 108, 116, 117, 122, 124
Antioxidants, 35, 44, 107, 117
Anxiety, 40, 45, 50, 54, 57, 58, 65, 74, 82, 87, 90, 99, 100, 101, 104, 106, 108, 116, 133, 136, 138, 156, 159

Anxiolytic, 34, 45, 46, 47, 128, 135, 144
Apoptosis, 57, 77, 118, 119, 128, 129, 130, 141, 159
Appetite, 21, 30, 31, 39, 40, 54, 63, 87, 103, 104, 114, 118, 128, 160
Arizona, 155
ASD, 101, 133, 134, 135, 136, 137, 138
Asthma, 65
Attention deficit hyperactivity, 26
Autism spectrum disorder, 57, 134, 136, 138
Autoimmune, 47, 65, 116, 154, 155, 156
Autoimmune diseases, 101, 116
Autophagic cell repair, 29
Basal ganglia, 25, 140
bhang tea, 62
Biden, Joe, 15
Bioavailability, 70, 71
Blood pressure, 24, 44, 73, 74, 75, 78, 89, 147
Bone growth, 39, 40, 101
Brain, 19, 21, 23, 24, 25, 26, 27, 42, 46, 49, 61, 68, 69, 73, 83, 103, 104, 110, 131, 136, 139, 140, 141, 160, 163
Brain Stem, 24
Brazil, 11, 127, 132
Breastfeeding, 84
Bronchial tree, 56, 61, 66
Bronchitis, 77
Bronchodilator, 46, 76
Bronchospasm, 74, 76
Bureau of Narcotics and Dangerous Drugs, 17
California, 2, 9, 10, 15, 32, 34, 59, 89, 114, 146, 147
Canada, 15, 61, 86
Cancer, 7, 9, 22, 29, 40, 47, 54, 57, 58, 65, 77, 78, 86, 100, 112, 113, 117, 124, 125, 128, 129, 130, 131, 154, 155, 159, 161, 163
Cannabene hydride, 34
Cannabichromene, 35, 39, 48

Cannabinoid, 7, 10, 11, 13, 19, 20, 21, 25, 26, 29, 30, 32, 34, 36, 37, 39, 40, 48, 55, 57, 63, 64, 69, 70, 71, 74, 79, 85, 99, 105, 110, 111, 114, 118, 119, 125, 126, 128, 129, 143, 144, 146, 147, 148, 151, 153, 154, 160, 161
cannabinoid acids, 64
Carcinogenic, 56, 66
Caryophyllene, 48
CB1, 19, 20, 21, 24, 25, 28, 31, 35, 41, 68, 69, 79, 84, 118, 125, 129, 136, 144, 158
CB2, 19, 20, 21, 25, 26, 31, 35, 41, 48, 79, 118, 125, 129, 144, 158
CBC, 35, 39, 43, 57, 110
CBCa, 37, 41, 43
CBD, 7, 27, 29, 30, 31, 32, 34, 35, 37, 40, 41, 43, 50, 54, 56, 57, 59, 60, 62, 63, 65, 67, 68, 71, 74, 78, 80, 81, 82, 89, 99, 110, 112, 123, 125, 126, 129, 131, 132, 133, 135, 137, 138, 142, 143, 147, 151, 152, 156
CBDa, 37, 41, 43, 62, 152
CBG, 35, 37, 43, 50, 57, 110, 125, 129, 152
CBN, 35, 37, 39, 43, 57, 110, 125, 129
CenCal Health, 146
Center for Medicinal Cannabis Research, 34, 114
Ceramide, 22
Cerebellum, 24
Cerebral cortex, 25, 139, 140, 141
Cesamet, 54, 91
Chemotherapy, 58, 70, 104, 130, 131
China, 7, 13, 14, 16, 74
Chlorophyll, 35
Citicoline, 82
Cognitive function, 27
Cole Memo, 15
Colorado, 15, 30, 155, 160
Contraindicationa, 9, 10, 94, 156
Cough, 65, 73, 74, 75, 76, 77
Courtney, William, 64
Crohn's disease, 11, 62, 101, 102, 116, 117, 118, 120, 155
Cultivar, 44, 81, 164
Cunha, 59, 132
Curran, Valerie, 83

Cytokines, 117, 119, 121, 142
Dabbing, 66, 160
Decarboxylation, 42, 160
Dependence, 8, 10, 51, 88, 89, 90, 92, 118
Dependency, 73, 88, 90, 164
Devitt-Lee, Adrian 29
Diabetes, 40, 100, 116
Diagnostic and Statistical Manual of Mental Disorders, 90, 91, 133
Digestion, 30
Dopamine, 25, 26
Dosage, 51, 52, 53, 55, 56, 57, 58, 60, 65, 66, 68, 81, 91, 99, 147, 152
Dowd, Maureen, 81
Dreher, Melody, 84
Dravet, 132, 137
Driving, 51, 73, 94, 95, 96
Drug Enforcement Administration, 17, 18
Drug interactions, 10, 69
Dysphoria, 55, 56, 57, 58, 60, 61, 62, 63, 64, 73, 80, 81, 82, 99, 160
Dysplasia, 65
Edibles, 62, 76
Egypt, 14
Eli Lilly, 17
Endocannabinoid system, 1, 3, 7, 9, 10, 11, 12, 18, 19, 21, 25, 26, 27, 29, 30, 83, 96, 97, 111, 136, 148, 149, 150, 151, 153
Endocannabinoids, 7, 19, 20, 25, 26, 74, 118, 119, 126, 128, 160
England, 14, 16, 59, 62, 132
Entourage effect, 48, 49, 50, 54, 63, 99, 161
Enzymes, 36
Epidiolex, 55, 61, 62, 132, 153
Epilepsy, 34, 41, 59, 60, 71, 99, 103, 105, 131, 132, 133, 137, 155
Euphoria, 31, 42, 54, 55, 56, 58, 63, 64, 68, 69, 80, 82, 89, 99, 160
Euphoriphobia, 54
Fatty acids, 36
FECO, 58, 61, 161, 164
Fibromyalgia, 32, 47, 155
Flavonoids, 35, 44, 50, 93, 152

France, 14
Free radicals, 29, 30, 163
Full extract cannabis oil, 58
Full spectrum, 48, 54, 60, 62, 63, 82, 153, 161, 162
Fungal infections, 43
G protein-coupled receptors, 25
Gastrointestinal tract, 21, 104, 116, 119
Glucose, 22, 40, 78, 101
Glutamate, 25, 26, 141
Goldstrich, Joe 58, 129, 155
Grinspoon, Lester, 49
Gut microbiome, 108, 122
GW Pharmaceuticals, 15, 34, 49, 59, 62, 63, 113, 129, 130
Harvard, 13, 34
Harvard University, 13
Hemp, 13, 17, 64, 129, 159, 162
Henningfield, Jack, 89
Herbalism, 10, 11
Hippocampus, 24
Hippocrates, 107, 108
HIV, 9, 70, 112
Homeostasis, 21, 22, 29, 30, 32, 129, 141, 160
Hydrocodone, 93
Hyperemesis, 64, 73, 79, 80, 162
Hypothalamus, 24
Ibuprofen, 82
Immune system, 21, 32, 43, 48, 116, 118, 123, 124
India, 7, 14, 16, 61, 62, 132
Indica, 34, 162
Inflammation, 21, 22, 31, 34, 41, 60, 78, 107, 116, 117, 118, 119, 123, 124, 125, 126, 131, 142, 143
Insomnia, 60, 103
Institute of Medicine, 74, 88, 113
Insulin, 22
Integrative, 48, 106, 107, 108, 158, 162
Investigational New Drug, 15, 52, 53
IQ, 73, 82, 83, 87
Irvine, 32, 114
Israel, 7, 14, 129, 154
Italy, 14

Jamaica, 84, 85, 87
Johns Hopkins, 17
Jones, Reese 89
Juicing, 62, 64
Ketones, 36
Lamers, C.T., 96
Lee, Martin, 27
Lennox-Gastaut, 70, 72, 132
Limbic system, 23
Limonene, 46, 47, 82
Linalool, 47
Lipids, 27, 68, 142
Lipogenesis, 22
Los Angeles, 114
Lou Gehrig's disease, 39
Macrophage, 79, 119, 123
Malka, Deborah 31, 57
Marihuana Tax Act, 14, 17, 18
Marijuana Research Center, 15
Marinol, 54, 55, 61, 63, 64, 91, 93, 147, 153
Mathre, Mary Lynn 53
Mechanisms of action, 10, 18, 148, 151
Mechoulam, 1, 3, 7, 8, 11, 19, 21, 25, 32, 34, 39, 40, 48, 49, 59, 99, 132, 137, 150, 151, 152, 154, 156, 157, 161
Medical review officers, 93
Meladmede, Robert 30
Merck, 17
Metabolic disorders, 40
Metabolism, 51, 67, 68, 70, 117
Methicillin-resistant Staphylococcus, 40
Mexico, 61, 67, 114, 159
Midbrain, 23, 25
Migraine, 14, 17, 26, 32, 55, 104
Minnesota, 114
Mitochondria, 27, 28, 29, 30, 32
Mood, 21, 30, 31, 139, 145
Multiple sclerosis, 58, 59, 105, 112, 116, 126, 155
Myrcene, 45, 49, 50
Nabilone, 54, 144
National Highway Traffic Safety Administration, 94, 95

Nausea, 17, 40, 54, 58, 64, 65, 79, 80, 87, 100, 104, 114, 116, 130, 131
Benowitz, Neal, 89
Neocortex, 23
Nervous tissue, 21
Neuralgia, 55
Neurotransmission, 22, 25, 26, 27, 33, 48, 110
Neurotransmitters, 25, 134, 142, 160
NIDA, 77, 78, 84, 85, 88, 89, 115
NORML, 21, 92, 115
Noyes, 56, 57, 113
Nutraceutical, 162, 163
Obama, Barack, 15
Ogden Memo, 15
Opioids, 71, 98, 111
Oregon Health and Sciences University, 66
O'Shaughnessy, 16, 132
Osler, 14, 17
Pain, 13, 26, 43, 47, 60, 71, 103, 108, 110, 111, 112, 113, 114
Panic attacks, 73, 102
Paranoia, 54, 58, 80
Parke-Davis, 17
Parkinson's disease, 40, 102
Patent medicines, 54
Peristalsis, 22
Peron, Dennis, 9
Persia, 14
Personalized medicine, 152
Phytocannabinoids, 19, 31, 35, 37, 118, 123, 129, 136, 142, 163
Phytol, 48
Piomelli, Danielle, 20, 25, 32, 33, 119
Pregnancy, 51, 83, 84, 85, 86, 87
Proposition 215, 9
Psoriasis, 43, 116, 120, 121, 122, 123, 124, 125, 126, 155
Psychosis, 43, 100
PTSD, 57, 73, 87, 90, 101, 102, 103, 154, 155
Pyrolysis, 53, 56, 66
Queen Victoria, 7, 17
Quercetin, 44
Jones, R.T., 78

Raw cannabis, 41, 53, 64, 65, 67
Reactive oxygen species, 29, 117, 141, 163
Reptilian Brain, 24
Rheumatoid arthritis, 40, 47, 62, 100, 116, 155
Rick Simpson Oil, 58, 161, 164
Routes of administration, 51, 61, 62, 147
Ruderalis, 164
Russo, 31, 35, 38, 39, 41, 42, 46, 47, 48, 49, 50, 53, 54, 98, 99
San Diego, School of Medicine, 34
San Francisco, 77, 89, 114, 129
Sativa, 104, 164
Sativex, 15, 55, 56, 57, 59, 61, 62, 63, 126, 127, 153
Schizophrenia, 100, 156
Scythia, 14
Seizure, 26, 40, 41, 59, 60, 63, 64, 65, 70, 72, 103, 104, 132, 133, 137
Serotonin, 25
Sharp and Dohme, 17
Shen Nung, 13, 16
Shultes, 13
Side effects, 7, 9, 10, 41, 49, 51, 54, 55, 57, 58, 63, 64, 70, 73, 74, 76, 80, 91, 95, 114, 118, 123, 136, 137, 144, 147, 149, 156
Sisley, Sue 155
Sleep, 30, 39, 40, 60, 74, 91, 99, 100, 103, 108, 118, 128, 136, 138, 160
Smith Brothers, 17
Smoking, 56, 61, 65, 75, 77
Spasticity, 39, 58, 59, 100, 116, 126
Sputum, 65, 74, 75, 76, 77, 116
Squibb, 17
Standardization, 62, 152, 153
Steffens et al., 79
Steroids, 36
Sublingual, 76
Substance abuse, 10, 91, 93
Sulak, Dustin, 57
Suppositories, 82, 164
Tachycardia, 73, 74, 76, 89, 99
Tashkin, Donald, 76, 77, 128
TBI, 73, 87, 103

Terpenes, 13, 35, 44, 45, 49, 50, 57, 61, 63, 66, 67, 77, 93, 99, 110, 130, 147, 148, 152, 165

THC, 7, 13, 22, 31, 34, 35, 37, 39, 41, 42, 43, 46, 47, 48, 49, 50, 52, 53, 54, 55, 56, 57, 58, 59, 60, 61, 62, 63, 64, 65, 66, 67, 68, 69, 71, 74, 75, 76, 79, 80, 81, 82, 83, 89, 91, 93, 94, 95, 96, 98, 99, 104, 110, 112, 113, 118, 120, 123, 125, 126, 128, 130, 136, 137, 138, 142, 143, 144, 147, 151, 152, 153, 158, 162, 163

THCa, 37, 41, 42, 43, 57, 62, 64, 152

THCV, 40, 43, 152

The Controlled Substances Act, 14

Tinctures, 62, 67, 76

Titration, 52, 164

Tolerance, 55, 91, 95

Topical, 61, 67

Torres, Ciara A., 84

Toxicology, 8, 10, 51, 69, 93

UN Single Convention on Narcotic Drugs, 14, 15, 146

Ungerleider, Thomas, 58, 59

United Kingdom, 15, 34, 54, 60

United Nations, 14

United States Pharmacopoeia, 14, 17

Uruguay, 15

US Department of Transportation, 93, 95

US Supreme Court, 14

USA, 14, 15

Vaping Associated Pulmonary Injury, 66

Vaporization, 56, 66, 76, 160

Vitamin E acetate, 66

Volcano, 66

Volkow, Nora, 115

Vomiting, 58, 74, 79, 80, 100, 104, 114, 130, 131, 162

Washington, 15, 77, 88, 95, 110, 111, 114, 133

Woodward, William 17, 18

About the Authors

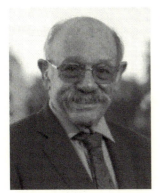

Dr. David Bearman received his M.D. from the University of Washington School of Medicine. He has served at all levels of government including the U.S. Public Health Service, Director of Health Services at San Diego State University, Health Officer and Director of Sutter County Health Department and Medical Director and Director of Medical Services for the Santa Barbara Regional Health Authority (now CenCal). He is the author of Drugs Are NOT the Devil's Tools.

Dr. Bearman has a long and illustrative half-century career in the field of drug abuse treatment and prevention. He was prominent in the community clinic movement, having started the third Free Clinic in the country in Seattle before directing the Haight Ashbury Drug Treatment Program, and in 1970 founding the Isla Vista Medical Clinic. He was Medical Director of Santa Barbara County Methadone Maintenance Clinic and Ventura County Opiate Detox Program, and Zona Seca, an outpatient drug treatment program.

He graduated from the University of Wisconsin in 1963 with a degree in Psychology and in 1967 obtained his M.D. degree from the University of Washington School of Medicine. He now maintains a private practice as a specialist in pain management and cannabinoid medicine in Goleta, California where lives with his wife, Lily (a career counselor). They have two adult children, Samantha and Benjamin.

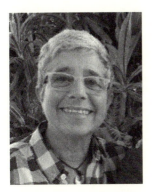

Maria Pettinato, RN, PhD, is an Associate Professor in the College of Nursing at Seattle University, Seattle, Washington. She is an experienced faculty member teaching Pathophysiology, Neurobiology, and Med/Surg nursing in both under-graduate and graduate programs on the east and west coast of the United States for the past 25 years. Her research interests focus on sexual minority health issues and medicinal cannabis. Her scholarly work focuses on substance use, mental health issues, and sexual minority health issues. She is the author of "Medicinal Cannabis: A Primer for Nurses."

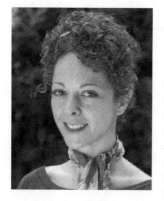

Dr. Carolina Nocetti is a clinician, educator, and technical consultant on medical cannabis projects in the United States, Canada, Uruguay, Paraguay, Colombia, Israel, and Brazil. She regularly testified in public hearings in Brazil, including in the Chamber of Deputies, Senate, and in the Legislative Assembly of the State of São Paulo. She is also the director of the international committee of the Pan-American Association of Cannabinoid Medicine (representing Brazil) and a member of the Advisory Council of the Parliamentary Front for Medical Cannabis in the Legislative Assembly of the State of São Paulo.

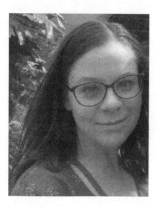

Angela Bacca has authored hundreds of articles and edited, managed, and/or co-authored over a dozen books, mostly on cannabis horticulture and medicine, in addition to editing and managing various cannabis-centric digital and print magazines. Her work has focused on cannabis economics, politics, science, horticulture, cultural issues, non-cannabis herbalism, and complementary and alternative health topics. She has been a legal medical cannabis patient diagnosed with an autoimmune disease for 20 years. She has a bachelor's degree in journalism from San Francisco State University and a master's in business administration from the Lorry I. Lokey Graduate School of Business at Mills College.